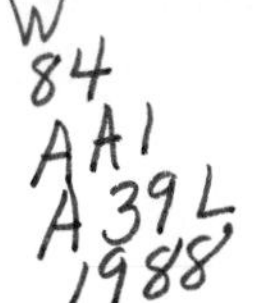

Contents

Preface

Health care in the 1990s will be vastly different than it is today. An aging poulation, the looming physician surplus, a changing federal role in health care, technological advances, and a plethora of new outpatient treatment facilities are all forcing changes in the nation's health care system.

In this report, the Institute for the Future (IFTF) of Menlo Park, California, singles out the trends most likely to change health care by describing differing scenarios of the system likely to emerge and by identifying the key choices that will face us by the year 2000.

The uncertainties around many of these changes led The Robert Wood Johnson Foundation and The Commonwealth Fund to support this three-year effort to generate a comprehensive picture of the evolution of the nation's health care system over the next thirteen years, including the likely implications for key health professional groups and for American society.

The goal of this project was to provide long-term planning assistance to health professional groups, private foundations, public and private sector decisionmakers involved in health care and, specifically, to four selected professional associations--the American Hospital Association, the American Medical Association, the Association of American Medical Colleges, and the Blue Cross and Blue Shield Association. This assistance was to include: (1) the identification of key environmental forces that are creating change in the American health care system to the year 2000; (2) the development of forecasts of the health care environment in the form of alternative scenarios; (3) the assessment of the impact of these changes on four key groups in the health care system (physicians, hospitals, academic medical centers, and health insurers); and (4) the identification of the major issues and choices likely to face private and public sector policymakers with regard to patient care in the year 2000.

From the beginning, we believed that in order for this study to be of genuine value to the professional associations, to their memberships, and to health policymakers in general, it was critically important that the associations and others who play a major role in the health care system be involved directly in the project. Their input would be essential in identifying key areas of concern; in specifying some of the broader social, technological, and economic forces that they thought would play a role in those areas; and in thinking through some of the issues likely to emerge for both health professionals and patients.

IFTF was thought to be uniquely suited to manage this ambitious undertaking. Established in 1968 as a nonprofit research organization, IFTF was one of the first research organizations dedicated to a systematic study of the long-term future. In its short life, it had earned a solid reputation for its efforts to link futures planning to practical decision making in private industry and government. In addition, IFTF had conducted an earlier study supported by The Robert Wood Johnson Foundation that had predicted a downturn in hospital admissions two years before the actual event occurred.

In the present study, IFTF served as both a facilitator and a resource. Working closely with the staffs of the professional associations and the two sponsoring foundations, it drew upon their expertise through a series of carefully structured workshops focusing on specific aspects of the future of health care.

IFTF also conducted a series of in-depth interviews with leading authorities in economics, government, technology, and public opinion to develop scenarios of the broader social context within which the health care system will operate over the coming decade.

As a means of ensuring the extensive involvement of the health professional groups, a steering committee was established that included high-level foundation and professional association officers in its membership. Robert Ebert, MD, former dean of Harvard Medical School and advisor to the presidents of The Robert Wood Johnson Foundation and The Commonwealth Fund, chaired the steering committee throughout its three-year life.

The collaboration of many distinguished professionals under the auspices of IFTF has resulted in a volume that is valuable to health professionals in a number of fields--and, most important, to concerned private and public decisionmakers who ultimately must set the future course of America's medical care.

Both the foundations and IFTF are deeply grateful to the many individuals who contributed their time and insights to developing this volume about medicine in the year 2000.

Robert J. Blendon
Senior Vice President
The Robert Wood Johnson Foundation
Princeton, New Jersey

Margaret E. Mahoney
President
The Commonwealth Fund
New York, New York

September 1987

Acknowledgments

This study would not have been possible without the special efforts of a number of individuals. The idea for the project was conceived jointly with Robert Blendon, senior vice president of The Robert Wood Johnson Foundation, as well as Thomas Moloney and Margaret Mahoney, senior vice president and president, respectively, of The Commonwealth Fund.

Robert Ebert, MD, advisor to the presidents of The Robert Wood Johnson Foundation and The Commonwealth Fund, provided the guiding hand in enlisting the cooperation of all participants, in cochairing all panel sessions, and in shepherding the project on a day-to-day basis. Paul Jellinek, senior program officer of The Robert Wood Johnson Foundation, gave us both strong intellectual and administrative support through direct participation in the many phases of the project.

Several IFTF staff members contributed substantially to the success of the study. Included were Mary Poulin, research fellow, who was involved in the early stages of study formulation and research; and Patricia Stern, Kathryn Lenihan, and Patricia Rogow, who were responsible for the production, illustration, and editing of the manuscript. Deborah Glazer, sponsoring editor at McGraw-Hill, guided us superbly through the process of publication.

Roy Amara, Project Director
J. Ian Morrison
Gregory Schmid
Institute for the Future
Menlo Park, California

May 1988

Overview: An Agenda for Health Care in the 1990s

The health care system in the United States is in turmoil as it goes through a period of radical structural changes. This study explores these changes and identifies impacts and issues for some key actors--physicians, hospitals, academic medical centers, and health insurers--and the society at large.

With the participation of approximately eighty nationally renowned experts[1], we identified the key driving forces that are likely to change the health care system by the year 2000. Utilizing those driving forces and the differing perceptions of the experts on how those forces would play out, we developed two alternative scenarios that provide plausible and internally consistent descriptions of the health care system. The scenarios were structured to capture the inherent and considerable uncertainties that exist in the possible evolution of health care (see Chapters 3 and 4). In developing the scenarios, we identified several key driving forces and major structural shifts in health care that are *common* to both scenarios. It is these "no matter what" characteristics of the health care system that are worthy of special attention. They set the stage for the critical issues and choices that are destined to loom large in the national debate on health care in the 1990s. Key driving forces, structural changes, and issues are presented here in distilled and summary form.

Key Driving Forces[2]

1. AGING

"With extended longevity we will see more and more people who survive multiple heart attacks and strokes. As a result, we will be faced with more people who don't know how to die and will become burdens to themselves and to the health care system."

---

[1]See Appendix A for a list of study participants.

[2]All quotes are drawn from statements made by study participants.

"This is a major factor since we are not facing up to the cost of health care delivery for an aging population. This group is physiologically making excessive demands on the health care system, and there is nothing on the horizon that will make costs diminish."

America is facing an explosion in the number of elderly, particularly in the over-75 population. The number of people over 75 will grow by almost 35 percent between 1985 and 2000. This group has historically been an extremely heavy user of health and hospital services--from five to seven times the average for the population as a whole. Even if the elderly of the future are healthier than their predecessors, the growth in the number of very old Americans will be a key driver of the system. At the extreme, the elderly could become an enormous burden on the nation's health care resources if we continue to apply all of the expensive technologies to this group. No matter what, the demands of the elderly, both medical and political, will be a key driving force for change. These pressures will be central to the policy debates on: funding and delivery of both Medicare and Medicaid; long-term care; home care versus institutional care; the use of technology; and the right-to-die.

2. SOPHISTICATED CONSUMERS

"The public has become more vocal and more knowledgeable about what it wants from the health care system. People read the stories about misdiagnosis and unnecessary surgery and are better consumers."

"Providers will be viewed less as high priests and more as professionals."

The baby boom represents the best educated cohort in America and is increasingly a group who will shape the health care system through their own interaction with the system and through their support for or opposition to health care policies. The elderly Americans of the 1990s also will be better educated than their predecessors and they too will represent a more sophisticated set of health care consumers than in the past. This sophistication will be felt in a number of ways. For example, consumers are less likely to treat providers as high priests and more as professionals, consumers will expect more of a role in medical decision making, and they will be a critical factor in the success of new delivery systems in a medical market that offers more and more choices.

3. PRESSURES FROM PAYERS

"The most important day in the health care field was the day that GM and Ford realized that health care costs were taking a larger share than expenditures for basic steel. Now all of industry has become aware of the problem."

"The health care system will be controlled more by payers than providers--with employers, consumers, and taxpayers exercising the greatest amount of power."

Between the mid-1960s and mid-1980s, government and business paid for increasing shares of health care costs. Those days are gone. Business will increasingly be concerned about the costs of health care as the pressures of global competition squeeze profits and make health benefits a more visible cost. Federal and state governments have to contend with high and increasing demands for services in areas such as health, education, and welfare, while antitax sentiment among the baby boom continues to build. The federal budget deficit is a key economic problem that will constrain spending through the 1990s. Consumers who have long been protected from the sting of health costs by third-party insurers will resist any efforts to place a major burden of payment on them. These three actors will resist cost expansion--how successful they will be is uncertain and this uncertainty represents the major difference between the two scenarios that will form the core of this volume. But whatever the outcome, the trend is clear--that the payers of the health care bill will be much more sensitive to economics and cost effectiveness during the 1990s.

4. PLURALISM AND DIVERSITY

"Our society more than any other is pluralistic. The most unified social policy of the United States has been social security--a national system applicable to everyone. But even here, fifty years later we have private pension plans, ESOPs, and IRAs because we don't believe in permitting a single system."

"As long as distinctions (within the health care system) are not based on poor versus rich, I say fine. If New York does one thing and North Dakota another, that's fine. But I don't think we would stand for a system where it was rich versus poor, where a Mississippi just could not afford the cost of care."

The U.S. health care system is a patchwork of public and private programs, state and federal government initiatives, and regional patterns of utilization and medical practice. The diversity of health care reflects the pluralism of American culture. A truly national health program on the British model is unlikely to materialize. Instead, the U.S. system will continue to be fractionated as state and regional health care systems of finance and delivery evolve to meet local market, political, and social needs.

5. TECHNOLOGICAL CAPABILITY

"Although technology has been reasonably important to health care in the last twenty years, it will have a major influence in the next twenty years. This is because we will just be at the turning point and we will have developed actual capabilities that will go beyond anything we can do now."

"It's not so much that we can expect brand new important technologies to be introduced in the next ten years; it's more a question of the pace of new innovations introduced into medical care. This will depend on the reimbursement system."

A wide set of new technologies are in the pipeline. They include drugs and devices, new techniques, and new approaches to diagnosis and treatment. Developments in the basic sciences, in computer and communications technology, and in our understanding of cellular mechanisms and the molecular biology of disease will lead to new medical technologies. The set of technologies is reasonably well known and will present incredibly tough choices about who gets access to these technologies and how we pay for them.

6. HEALTH CARE CAPACITY

"More doctors means more trouble and we will have doctors coming out of our ears. More doctors will find patients . . . It is not possible to affect the number of doctors significantly in the next ten to fifteen years even if some medical schools were closed today."

"With an excess of beds and doctors, insurers and business are getting deals with providers and this is shifting activity."

The number of physicians in the United States will continue to rise until the end of the century. The doubling in the annual number of new physicians that took place in the 1960s has left a legacy of excess capacity that will remain over the balance of this century and into the next. Whether this continued increase will lead to greater competition or to greater per capita utilization depends on choices, both public and private, that will be made over the next decade. Similarly, as hospital admissions and length-of-stay decline or grow more slowly than historically, empty hospital beds are likely to persist as a problem almost everywhere. What is not so clear is how this overcapacity will affect long-run health care costs.

7. HEALTH CARE GROWTH

"Needs will increase, and unless we ignore these needs, we are unlikely to keep costs down."

"We don't know what the top limit will be. If the prospect of increased longevity is correct, why would the ratio of health care expenditures to GNP stop at even 20 percent?"

The health care industry in the United States is headed upward. Although there is disagreement about how fast, the consensus seems to be that health care expenditures will at the very least keep pace with growth in the economy as a whole. For the expected range of economic growth through the 1990s, this translates into a minimum real growth rate of between 2 percent and 3 percent per annum through the balance of the century. If cost containment practices are not successful, then we can reasonably expect real growth rates of between 4 percent and 5 percent. Health care is a growth business compared to many other sectors of the U.S. economy because "people want more" and they are inclined to pay more if necessary.

8. GOVERNMENT AS STEERING AGENT

"In contrast (to the general trend toward deregulation) in those areas where the government is a big purchaser, it is regulating more. Health care is a prime example."

"Government will keep pressure on cost containment but will also tell people how to do things. They will continue to redefine what they pay for and how much they will pay. Talk will be of competition, but it's actually a more regulated system. More directions will be set: laws that mandate without necessarily paying (for example, risk pools for the uninsured, standards of care set for hospitals, and so forth)."

The government will continue to play a critical role in U.S. health care both as payer and as rulemaker. Efforts set in motion under the Reagan Administration have been designed to encourage competition in health care and to encourage premium funded rather than trust funded benefits. This trend will continue. But, in addition, government at federal, state, and local levels will be setting directions for the system by requiring other actors to behave a certain way or to pay for certain programs. The resolution of problems of cost, quality, and access will involve government as a steering agent.

Structural Shifts in Health Care (1985 versus 2000)

1. GROWTH OF MANAGED CARE

At a minimum, managed care will almost double, with coverage rising from 18 percent to 33 percent of total population.

The cost containment pressures of the mid- and late 1980s are acting as spurs for experimentation and innovation in health care delivery forms. Even if the system continues to expand the range of services it provides, the capitated and contract sectors will almost double in size (in terms of population covered) from 1985 to 2000. Managed care will then extend to at least one-third of the total population and possibly to over one-half. Capitated plans in particular will grow in popularity because enrollees will perceive them as providing better value (wider range of covered services), not just less expensive health care. The most successful plans in enrolling customers will not be the fully integrated types of providers such as staff-model HMOs, but capitated plans negotiated with a series of physician groups and hospitals.

2. SALARIED PHYSICIANS UP, AUTONOMY DOWN

The percentage of salaried nonresident physicians will at least double between 1985 and 2000.

As the number of active physicians increases, so does the number of salaried physicians. By the year 2000, the percentage of nonresident patient care physicians who are on salary will almost double from 9 percent of the total to at least 17 percent and possibly to as high as 35 percent of the total. This is because many new physicians--particularly the more than 40 percent of new graduates that are women--prefer salaried positions, where an employer assumes the overhead costs and the economic risks of practice. For the more likely circumstances in which prepaid care grows somewhat more rapidly, the growth of salaried physicians will be even greater--to as much as 35 percent of nonresident physicians by 2000. In this instance, growth of salaried physicians will be enhanced by the move of many older physicians from active practice to research and administrative positions.

Under either circumstance, physicians--whether self-employed or not--will face some reduction in autonomy from the 1980s. The increasing emphasis on both consumer sovereignty and insurer oversight will lead to some reductions in clinical autonomy (the freedom to select treatments and styles of practice) and somewhat larger reductions in economic control (equipment purchases, price setting, and so forth). Still, the daily activity pattern of many physicians will remain largely unchanged. A substantial number of self-employed physicians will derive some of their income from contract or capitated care systems through a part-time salaried position. Also, many who work on hospital staffs or in professionally managed groups may receive a portion of their incomes on a fee-for-service basis through some HMO or PPO participation.

3. HOSPITAL ADMISSIONS "DOWN BUT NOT OUT"

Hospital admissions in the year 2000 will be at least 90 percent of their 1985 level.

Under the worst of circumstances for hospitals, total patient days will decline by 30 percent between 1980 and 1990 and then rebound in the late 1990s as the aging population makes itself felt. By 2000, the total days of hospital care will not decline by more than 10 percent from 1985 levels. The drop in activity is a phenomenon that will affect all age groups, with a slightly sharper fall for the under-65 age group. The rate of admissions per person in the population over 65 is about 3.5 times as high as the population under 65. In these circumstances--because of the more rapid growth in the number of people over 65--admissions of those over 65 will rise from 29 percent in 1985 to 35 percent of all admissions in 2000.

Under more favorable conditions for hospitals, admissions will stabilize earlier and rebound earlier, edging up about 10 percent in the year 2000 over 1985 levels. In either case, however, it will become apparent that economic failure is inevitable for some community hospitals unless some beds are taken out of service or converted.

4. SHIFT TO AMBULATORY ENVIRONMENT

Hospital outpatient activities will grow from levels of about 16 percent to at least 25 percent of total income.

The decline in hospital inpatient activities will go hand-in-hand with the rapid growth of hospital outpatient services. Included here are on-site outpatient activities such as ambulatory care facilities and outpatient testing as well as off-site functions that support and provide ancillary services to other local health care deliverers, sponsored HMOs or associated PPOs, community imaging centers, and testing laboratories. By the year 2000, such outpatient activities will grow from levels of about 16 percent of all hospital income in 1985 to at least 25 percent by the year 2000. Thus, while hospital buildings will be less central to the health care delivery system than they were, hospital administrators will continue to be deeply involved in almost every aspect of community health delivery.

5. INCREASE IN INTENSITY OF INPATIENT CARE

Inpatient expenditures per acute care admission will rise from $3,300 to about $5,000 (in constant 1985 dollars).

Length-of-stay has declined steadily from 8.2 days in 1970 to 7.1 days in 1985. No further reduction in hospital stays will occur from the current level of about 7 days per hospital admission. As a result of cost containment pressures and the organizational styles hospitals have adopted, some further slight reduction in length-of-stay may be expected until the early 1990s. Beyond that period, however, as more care is moved to outpatient settings and as the hospital population ages even more rapidly than total population, a rebound in length-of-stay may be expected.

The hospital of the 1990s will represent a core of high-intensity, high-technology care. The intensity, sophistication, and cost of inpatient care will increase dramatically as measured by expenditures per acute care admission--rising from about $3,300 in 1985 to about $5,000 in 2000. This is because patients that are less seriously ill will be spun off into ambulatory clinics or separate nursing units. One consequence of this shift will be a shortage of critical care staff in the hospital--particularly nurses and other allied health workers who are likely to seek more lucrative and less stressful work elsewhere.

6. DECLINE IN MEDICAL SCHOOL APPLICANTS

Applicants to U.S. medical schools will decline between 6 percent and 18 percent.

The decline in applicants to medical schools reflects two over arching trends: first, the demographic reality of the baby-bust generation of the late 1960s and 1970s who represent a smaller demographic pool of potential applicants; second, the wide-spread belief that too many physicians had been produced and that the rate of production should at least level off if not decrease. The result will be a decline in medical school enrollments of at least 6 percent and perhaps by as much as 18 percent by the year 2000.

However, even under the most adverse circumstances for medical schools, continuing strong public support for health care will make it extremely difficult politically for any state to close down an existing public medical college. At most, a few will consolidate and no new medical colleges will open. Under the press of declining applicant numbers, medical schools will find it makes more sense to reduce the sizes of incoming classes than to allow the applicant/acceptance ratio to fall much below what is considered a minimum (1.7). The leveling off in both the application rate and the applicant/acceptance ratio implies that there is no significant decline in the quality of students.

7. INCREASING CONCENTRATION OF MEDICAL RESEARCH DOLLARS

The top twenty medical schools will increase their share of research funding from 50 percent to 56 percent.

Even under the most adverse circumstances, the income of medical schools will continue to expand in real terms--at least at half of the growth rate of total health care spending. On the research side, however, the distribution of research dollars for medical schools will become even more skewed. As private sources of research funding become even more prominent, more money will be channeled to the larger and better funded schools and departments. Even expanding (NIH) budgets will be allocated increasingly to favor particular academic institutions as the feeling grows that they are the best bets in the race for the United States to maintain world leadership in medical technology. Thus, whereas the top twenty elite medical schools accounted for 50 percent of all research funding in 1985, by 2000 they will account for 56 percent of the total.

8. GROWTH IN COST OF PROGRAM ADMINISTRATION AND NET COST OF INSURANCE

The cost of program administration and net cost of health insurance will increase by at least 70 percent in real dollars.

However the health care system evolves--toward more contract and capitated care or toward a complex hybrid system of managed and fee-for-service care--the cost of program administration and the net cost of health insurance will increase by at least 70 percent (in constant 1985 dollars) between 1985 and the year 2000. This net cost includes the administrative costs of public and private sector insurance and profits flowing to for-profit organizations.

In an environment of rapidly growing contract and capitated care, the costs of managing the more complex contracts is high as benefit administrators demand more information on the care administered, the costs of each element of that care, and measures of quality of that care. In addition, providers will spend more time in administration, controlling their own costs, and developing data on the quality of care being provided.

Alternatively, in a more market-driven environment, many new insurance products are diffused through the health care system: long-term care coverage, "boutique" products such as coverage for certain occupations, and so on. The spread of cafeteria plans and individualized "wellness" premium rebates virtually spell the end of traditional group contracts with their lower unit costs. Again, it costs more to manage care.

Fifty Critical Issues and Choices

The transformation in the structure of the health care system will change the role of some key stakeholders, and the threats and opportunities they face will force them to confront some critical choices.[1] Here we summarize the choices faced by five such stakeholders: physicians, hospitals, academic medical centers, health insurers, and the larger society.[2]

PHYSICIANS

The decade of the 1990s will be a turbulent one for physicians. The number of physicians rises dramatically as current medical school graduates move into active practice. The greater proportion of females among young physicians and medical school students increases their relative share of practicing physicians over the period. The number of young physicians in salaried jobs increases. The expenses associated with running a physician's office rise dramatically over the period, putting a greater priority on financial controls. But most of all, physicians undergo a loss of autonomy and independence as responsibility for care must be shared increasingly with payers, insurers, and patients. The major issues and implications for physicians in the 1990s are summarized below:

1. Physician surplus: growing competition for customers.

2. Physician autonomy: growing constraints on physician's economic and clinical decisionmaking.

3. Practice styles: increasing physician responsiveness to payer standards.

4. Physician/hospital relationships: shifting of power away from physicians toward hospitals.

5. Physician/government relationships: conflicting pressures on physicians from government for cost effectiveness *and* quality.

6. Rationing of care: diminishing role and shared decisionmaking of physicians in critical patient care choices.

---

[1]See Appendix B for a description of study methodology, including how the issues and choices were generated.

[2]See Chapters 5 through 9 for a detailed description of these issues and choices.

7. End-of-life care: increasing physician confrontation with ethical and moral choices.

8. Malpractice: continuing cost and practice burden for physicians in independent practices.

9. Role of medical associations: growing need to redefine roles and missions.

HOSPITALS

Perhaps more than any other major health care stakeholder, hospitals find themselves at the center of change no matter where they turn. Hospital admissions grow very slowly--when they grow at all--as increasing emphasis is placed on the ambulatory care environment. The intensity of inpatient care increases dramatically as the hospital becomes the locus of care for the very sick. Competition between hospitals and other delivery systems and between hospitals and physicians intensifies. In addition, there is no let-up in the increasing pressures to consolidate and improve the efficiency of the small independent and underutilized hospital. The key threats and opportunities facing hospitals are summarized below:

1. Hospital competition: changing from competition for prestige to competition for survival.

2. Dependence on government: growing dependence of hospitals on government revenues.

3. Appropriate size/appropriate mission: declining inpatient utilization forcing a return to fundamentals.

4. Limits of diversification: emerging new competitors limit wide excursions from "home base."

5. Mergers and closures: increasing loss of some small (under 100-bed) hospitals creating hardships in rural areas.

6. Capital: growing limits on access to capital.

7. Openness and depth of review: increasing legal challenges to use of hospital cost and quality data.

8. Hospital/physician confrontation: increasing conflicts between hospitals and physicians in control of patients, technology acquisition, and pattern of care.

9. Uncompensated care: increasing pressure on government to resolve growing burden of uncompensated care on hospitals.

10. Effective use of medical technology: growing emphasis on technology assessment and regionalization of technology.

11. Acuity, staffing, and burnout: rising wages for acute inpatient care.

12. Hospital automation: growing need for capital intensiveness of the hospital.

ACADEMIC MEDICAL CENTERS

Medical schools--particularly those not in the top tier--will face some severe challenges in adapting to the world of the 1990s. Each will be faced with a decline in the demographic pool of medical school applicants, a reduction in the length of post-graduate education, an increase in the concentration of research dollars in the elite schools, a greater problem for teaching hospitals in keeping their share of the outpatient market, and continued reliance on the activities of the university's own resources. The specific issues confronting medical schools in the 1990s include:

1. Paying for medical education: growing financial pressures on some second-tier schools.

2. Clinical/academic trade-offs: increasing conflicts between academic and service objectives.

3. Town and gown: growing contentiousness between faculty and nonfaculty physicians.

4. Medical school curriculum: growing tensions on appropriate locus for clinical experience.

5. Medicine and other health professionals: increasing conflicts between medical schools and schools of nursing, social work, dentistry, pharmacy, public health, and so forth.

6. Women in medicine: growing numbers of women in medicine affecting the supply of nurses and the practice style and cost of medicine.

7. Funding of biomedical research: changing national priorities in funding of research versus funding of development.

8. Commercialization of science: increasing tensions and blurring boundaries between industry and academia on the free flow of new knowledge.

9. Clinical researchers: growing need to revitalize the role of the MD clinical researcher.

10. Fragmentation and tiering in academic medicine: growing disparities among medical schools in quality of programs and access to subspecialty training.

PRIVATE HEALTH INSURERS

The large traditional insurance firms do well after the threats of the 1980s. They continue to take advantage of the economies of scale they have as well as their ability to organize and manage information technology and to utilize experienced management, pricing experience, access to capital, and widespread local presence. The more effective management of insurance firms stops the trend to self-insure. However, the growth in managed care creates a more adversarial role between insurers and providers. It also brings insurers into the foreground in managing quality by ensuring that cost containment policies are not taken too far. As a result, the cost of administration remains high for both public and private insurers, taking a higher share of total health care dollars in the United States than in most other industrial countries. More specifically, the following issues and implications confront insurers in the 1990s:

1. New markets: growing opportunities for new products and services to meet mandated coverage and diminished or changed role of government as insurer.

2. Insurer/provider relationships: rethinking of positioning strategies for insurers.

3. Complexity of contracting: expanding the range and flexibility of benefit packages being offered.

4. Paying for vulnerable groups: redefining the boundaries of responsibility between public and private sector insurance.

5. Quality and insurers: increasing responsibility of insurers as prime guarantors of quality.

6. Tax and antitrust policies: levying of new taxes by government on health insurance and withdrawing nonprofit status of Blue Cross and Blue Shield organizations.

7. Ethical conflicts: increasing ethical conflicts for insurers in dealing with payers, providers, and patients.

8. Cultural change among the Blues: changing status of traditional quasi-public Blue Cross and Blue Shield organizations requires drastic staff and management shifts.

PUBLIC POLICY

The overarching public policy issue in health care in the 1990s is cost containment and how it should be approached. No national consensus exists on the preferred approach and, indeed, on whether to contain costs at all. A number of subsidiary public policy issues are derivative from this basic dilemma. For example, quality becomes a major public policy focus in both scenarios but for different reasons; ethical and economic choices surrounding the use of technology become more difficult in both scenarios; and health status and prevention continue to improve in both scenarios, albeit at slightly different rates. Looming large also is access to health care for specific vulnerable groups--the uninsured, the elderly in long-term care, mothers and children, and those with AIDS. The eleven issues that are likely to dominate the national health care agenda are summarized below:

1. Controlling costs: continuing contentiousness and conflict between various actors in health care; tough choices by government, business, labor, and families; acrimonious public debate.

2. Uninsured and underinsured: continuing problem with uninsured and underinsured requires federal, state, and local governments to develop more coherent policies for high-risk groups.

3. Long-term care: expanding debate over public/private insurance roles and responsibilities, limiting progress on financing and delivering long-term care.

4. Mother-child: continuing health needs of this group requires increased coordination and cooperation of both medical and social interventions.

5. AIDS: emerging health crisis raises fundamental questions about the role of government in health care insurance, financing, and regulation.

6. Quality in a competitive environment: measuring, managing, and assuring quality supplanting cost as key issues in the next decade.

7. Health manpower: raising questions about adequacy of the flow of trained personnel to meet future health care needs.

8. Health R&D: requiring sustained research and development focusing on potential high-impact areas.

9. Redeploying capital: increasing reliance on market forces to determine where new facilities will be located and who will get new equipment.

10. Tort liability: increasing role of courts in setting standards for care at all levels.

11. Ethics: raising a host of questions on roles and responsibilities as well as conflicts of interest for individuals practitioners, the professions, and society.

Introduction

Study Process[1]

Our general objective in this study was to identify the critical issues facing key stakeholders in the health care system through the use of scenarios--plausible and comprehensive pictures of the future system. These issues were generated by those most knowledgeable about, or most directly involved in, the workings of that system. The role of IFTF and the foundations was to structure, orchestrate, and distill the judgments of those individuals invited to participate in the study.

The sponsoring foundations enlisted the cooperation of four participating national organizations (PNOs) to facilitate access to representative individuals from physician, hospital, academic medical center, and insurer groups. The PNOs were: American Medical Association, American Hospital Association, Association of American Medical Colleges, and Blue Cross and Blue Shield Association.[2] At the outset, these groups were instrumental in helping to frame the study, to define a set of key descriptors of health care of most interest to each group, and to identify those factors external to health care that were most important in shaping the health care system. But in our view, an important part of the rationale underlying the selection of these four groups was to help foster and encourage basic institutional changes for these groups--institutional changes that must proceed hand in hand with the restructuring of health care.

The selected external factors (state of the economy; demography; households and lifestyles; attitudes; role of government; and technology) became the "grist" for constructing our environmental scenarios. The forecasts embedded in our scenarios were generated through one-on-one personal interviews with a carefully selected group of nationally renowned individuals[3] whose expertise was specifically matched to the factors. IFTF used the forecasts--including the perceived interactions among forecasts--provided by the experts to construct two plausible, internally consistent environmental scenarios.

---

[1]A detailed description of the study process appears in Appendix B.

[2]No endorsement of study findings by these organizations is intended or implied.

[3]See Appendix A for a list of study participants.

These scenarios provided the "backdrop" for representatives from the four PNOs to generate forecasts of structural changes in the health care system, to assess impacts on each group, and to identify issues and choices likely to be confronted by group members. Each group (for example, physicians, hospital administrators, academic medical center directors, and insurers) was assembled twice for full-day working sessions. In the first session, they were led through a process for making provisional forecasts of descriptors they had selected (for example, physician income, hospital admissions, number of medical schools, percent population in capitated care). These forecasts were predicated on assumptions about the external environment contained in our two environmental scenarios. Thus, in a real sense, the groups constructed "extensions" of our environmental scenarios into the health care system.

In the second session, we provided each group with distilled versions of the two alternative pictures contained in their provisional forecasts as well as forecasts made by the other three groups. This time, each group adjusted, modified, and balanced its provisional forecasts. At the same time, we asked each group to identify a set of health care issues--threats, opportunities, and choices. In particular, members of the group were asked to identify issues that were evoked by one or both scenarios. In some cases, the scenarios amplified the concern about a specific issue that was currently on the agenda of the group--for example, a surplus of physicians or hospital competition. In other cases, the scenarios helped the group highlight new issues--for example, decline of clinical and economic autonomy of physicians as a result of the increase in managed care.

In the final phase of the study, a public policy panel of distinguished generalists was convened. The objective was twofold: to review and critique the forecasts and health care issues, and to identify a set of public policy issues that were related to but distinct from the health care issues generated by representatives of the PNOs, using an issue-generation process similar to that used for the PNOs.

During the course of the study, a number of other individuals and organizations were drawn into the study to provide more depth and balance. Included were representatives from commercial insurers, business, government, and labor. The forecasts, impacts, and issues contained in this report are truly a composite of a wide range of individual viewpoints, perceptions, and judgments drawn from outside the sponsoring foundations and IFTF.

Developing the Scenarios

An important part of this study was to develop scenarios that distilled the perceptions of the participants. The study was not designed to develop normative visions of what the health care system ought to be like, nor was it designed to present extreme views of the health care system in the future. The selection of the participating national organizations and the external experts and, indeed, the design of the process itself were intended to develop views of the emerging health care system that were credible to the groups who would be using the information. The scenarios that have emerged span the range of the most plausible outcomes expected by the vast majority of the study participants. The results may seem somewhat conservative to readers who might view scenarios as spanning the range of possible outcomes and thus might have expected more radical departures from the present. But such radical departures-- for example, National Health Insurance on the British or even Canadian model, a massive reorientation of the health care system toward prevention and less intensive medical care, or complete privatization of the health care system--were not seen as highly likely given the political, organizational, and economic context of the United States in the 1990s.

The scenarios are not mutually exclusive. A variety of alternatives could be constructed using elements of both.[1] The reader is not asked to accept either scenario as an independent forecast or prediction; rather, taken together, they represent a point of departure for asking questions about health care issues and choices, for testing alternative strategies, and for identifying the possible effects of key trends on a variety of actors.

Scenarios are logical descriptions of plausible futures. Given that the future is by definition uncertain, a key step in generating scenarios is determining how many scenarios will be used to span the range of uncertainty about the future and how those scenarios should be structured. The primary reason for developing these two particular scenarios is that the input we received from the interviews with experts (see Appendix B on study process) yielded two recognizable clusters of responses. Experts were presented with a range of outcomes (four possible ranges of health care spending as a share of GNP) and asked to develop the logic underlying the development of that outcome, the driving forces involved, and the likelihood of this outcome occurring. The experts tended to collapse the four alternatives to two--each having support from approximately half of the respondents. One group of experts was confident that the forces for cost containment and rationalization in health care had sufficient momentum to affect the long run growth in costs; the other cluster provided evidence that, despite any efforts to restrain the system, the underlying forces for growth were more powerful. In capsule form, the two scenarios are:

---

[1]See Appendix C--How to Use the Study.

Scenario I: Tough Choices. This scenario presents a health system that is driven by cost containment pressures in which managers play an increasingly important intermediary role between payers and providers. The key change in the structure of the health care delivery system is a decline in the use of fee-for-service and growth in the contract and capitated sectors. This world of cost containment and managed care favors payers--business, government, and consumers--but has less palatable effects on providers, the disadvantaged working poor, and the medically indigent. At the same time, from a societal perspective, the health care system is well positioned to weather the economic storm when the baby boom hits retirement. The system is indeed lean.

Scenario II: Health and Wealth. This scenario presents an alternative and equally plausible view of the future in which the needs and wants of an increasingly affluent and technologically sophisticated society lead to a wider range of services aggressively marketed through hybrid financing and delivery mechanisms. Service expansion is characterized by the increased clout of consumers, more generous reimbursement than in the cost containment years, and an increasing role by multi-unit providers. This system also has its problems: the misuse of technology, the unnecessary duplication of facilities and services, and high and rising costs of health care before the real crunch when the baby boomers reach retirement.

Common Characteristics

The bulk of this report focuses on the two scenarios of the health care delivery system through the 1990s. The scenario format allows us to focus on the critical uncertainties that separate forecasts and to explore the impacts of different forecasts on the key actors. Still, it is important to note that virtually any forecast of the health care system shares some important common characteristics. In some cases, these common characteristics are also important driving forces shaping change in any scenario--for example, the aging of the population, the emergence of new technologies, or the continued thrust of U.S. society toward pluralism and diversity. In other cases, these characteristics are simply background assumptions that are not explicitly stated in the scenarios, because they do not help the reader differentiate between the scenarios--for example, population growth and changes in disease states.

DEMOGRAPHIC

Population growth will slow in the United States from an average of over 1 percent per year in the early 1980s to around 0.7 percent per year in the late 1990s. Total population will reach 274 million people in the year 2000. The number of elderly (those 65 years of age and over) will increase substantially, from 28.5 million in 1985 to 35 million in 2000. At the same time, the largest single cohort will be the baby boom cohort--those people born between 1945 and 1965 who will be between the ages of 35 and 55 in the year 2000.

ECONOMIC

The basic economic forces point to a moderate economic growth rate. A nation's long-term economic growth rate is approximately equivalent to the sum of the rate of growth of the work force and the productivity of its work force. Countries at the edge of the technology frontier have been able to sustain productivity growth rates of about 2 percent per year. Since work force growth will be less than 1 percent per year to the end of the century, real economic growth rates in the United States will average between 2.5 percent and 3 percent per year between 1986 and 2000. The moderate rates of economic growth and the current scale of the government's budget deficit imply that it will take a substantial effort to reduce the deficit. The process of working the deficit down almost inevitably means that taxes will increase without major expansions in government programs.

TECHNOLOGY

The basic thrust of American (and world) technology will continue over the time frame, regardless of scenario differences. The funding for basic R&D may vary slightly between scenarios, but the underlying innovative thrusts in medical technologies--information systems and biotechnology--will be very similar in either scenario.[1] In both scenarios, there will be a continuous flow of new drugs and progressive implementation of new information systems by both payers and providers. What is important for the delivery of health care is the relative rates of the diffusion of technology--what types of technologies will be used by whom and in what settings. It is the relative rate of diffusion of specific types of technologies that separates the two scenarios.

---

[1]See Appendix D--Important Technologies: Selected Candidates for Change.

DIVERSITY

The scenarios focus on key trends and macro indicators of change. Neither dwells on describing the persisting regional and local texture of the U.S. health care delivery system--a diverse blend of practice styles in a variety of geographic settings with important differences in regional and state rules and regulations. State-mandated reimbursement will be just as different between California and New Jersey in 2000 as it was in 1985. The difference in practice style between an inner city community clinic and a suburban group practice office will be wider than any differences described in the two scenarios. The American health care system will continue to experience this enormous diversity within the context of the macro changes described in the two scenarios.

DISEASE STATES

By the year 2000, cardiovascular diseases, cancer, and age-related problems are likely to remain the leading health problems in the United States (and in other developed countries). The "new kid on the block"--and fourth on the list--is Acquired Immune Deficiency Syndrome (AIDS).[1]

Few diseases can compare in speed and potential severity of impact with the onset of AIDS. From the *initial* perception by our experts and the PNO participants that AIDS was a wild card to be watched very closely, it has very quickly captured the public "spotlight" as no other health issue has in recent times. It has now become increasingly clear that AIDS will remain high on the public health agenda for years to come. Without some breakthrough advance in AIDS prevention or treatment, the following estimates have been made: by the end of the century, new cases of AIDS can range from an average of 125,000 per year to 500,000 per year, with cumulative cases numbering between 1 million and 3.6 million, respectively.[2]

---

[1]The Bristol Myers Report, "Medicine in the Next Century," Louis Harris and Associates, 1987.

[2]The Bristol Myers Report, "Medicine in the Next Century," Louis Harris and Associates, 1987.

THE UNEXPECTED

The future is shaped by two types of processes: underlying trends and specific events. Scenarios are constructed primarily using key trends and the uncertainty surrounding those trends. But there also are likely to be events that cannot be linked in any logical way to particular conditions or environmental areas such as the economy or demography. The term "wild card" is used to describe events that could have a major impact on the health care system but that are considered to be of low probability.

A series of wild cards was identified both from the interviews with experts on which the environmental scenarios are based and from the second round of workshops with PNO participants. Because these events are of low probability, neither scenario is predicated on their occurrence. But they raise a number of very interesting possibilities that should be considered in any contingency planning activities by major actors and policymakers.

The wild cards fall into five categories: (1) changes in technology; (2) changes in the organization of health care; (3) changes in epidemiology; (4) shifts in the role of government; and (5) other external events. The complete list of wild cards is shown in Appendix E.

Scenario 1: Tough Choices

Overview

Efforts to control health care costs finally come to fruition in the mid- and late 1980s. After almost two decades of rapid escalation--health care costs rose from 5.9 percent of GNP in 1965 to 10.7 percent in 1985--a strong societal consensus emerges that effective action is needed to constrain costs. This consensus is sustained by the relatively young college educated baby boom group that has family concerns on its mind; the competitive climate--both domestically and internationally--for business; the concern of the government over budget deficits; and the public's sharp eye on the public purse and the family budget. By the year 2000, total health care expenditures as a percent of GNP remain at their 1985 level, though the actual dollar figure rises from $425 billion in 1985 to $622 billion (in 1985 dollars) in 2000 (see figure 1).

Figure 1
U.S. Health Care Spending (As a Percent of GNP)

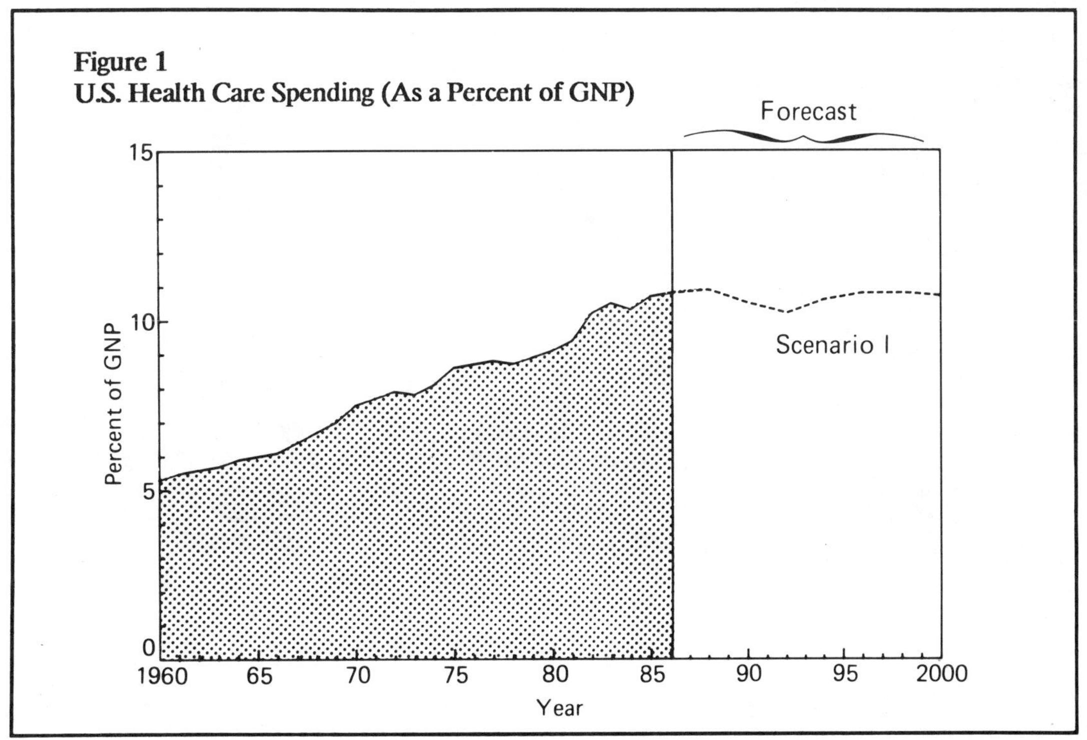

Forces for Containment

DEMOGRAPHIC FORCES: THE BABY BOOM'S ACTIVE YEARS

A keystone to the changes of the next decade is the aging of America. The share of population over 65 increases from 12 percent in 1985 to 13 percent in 2000. But of even more importance is the maturing of the baby boomers. This cohort, born between 1945 and 1965, is so large that it has always had a major impact in defining the dominant societal attitudes. By 1990, this group is between 25 and 45 years old and accounts for 33 percent of the total population (see figure 2). In 1980, 25 to 45 year old accounted for less than 28 percent of the population. From the 1980s up to the mid-1990s, the prime concerns of the baby boomers are purchasing a house, forming a family, educating and caring for their children, advancing their career paths, establishing a role in the community, and securing their personal financial position. It is also the time of life when health concerns are minimal, involving primarily preventive care and routine childhood illnesses.

Figure 2
Changing U.S. Age Distribution

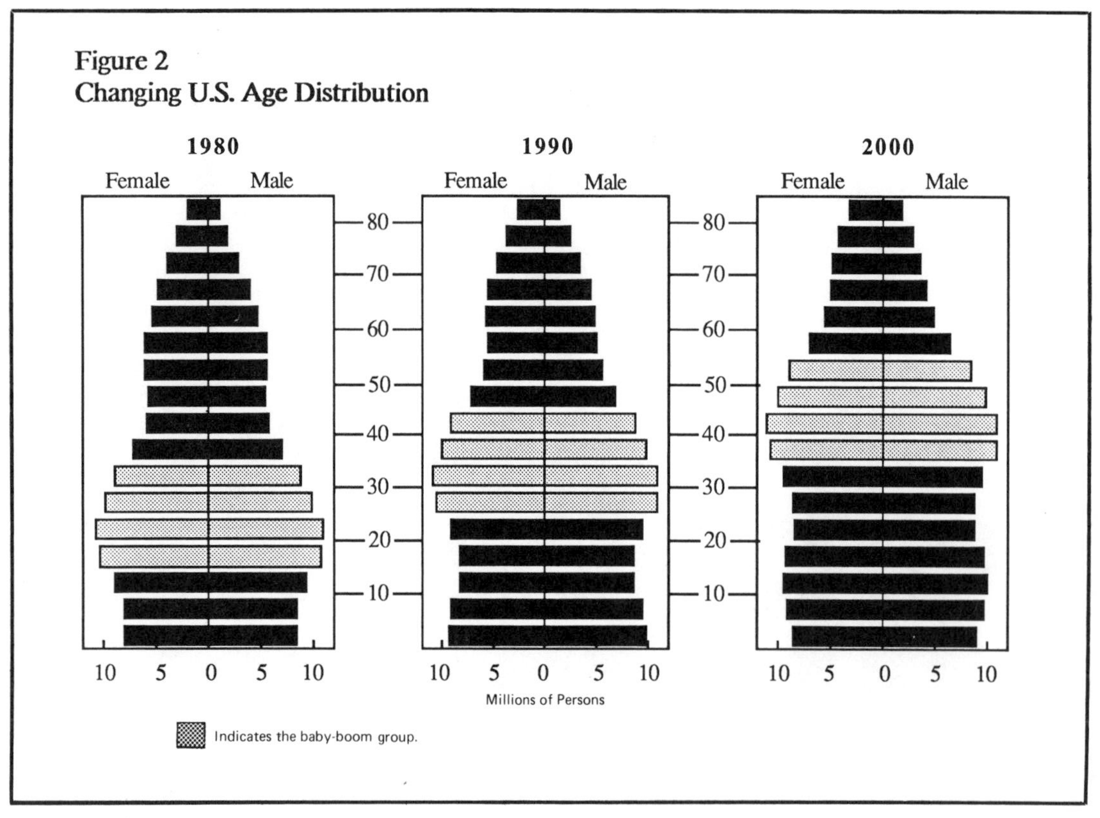

These stage-of-life characteristics mean that--at least until the late 1990s--this large cohort is in a traditional debtor position, borrowing to finance homes, household durables, education, and even vacations. Because of its debtor position, this dominant group is especially sensitive to increases in inflation, interest rates, and taxes. By the late 1990s, as the group moves from net debtors to net savers, its financial concerns ease to some extent as discretionary income rises. It is only at this time that the strong anti-tax spirit that became so prevalent in the mid-1980s begins to wane and public policy proposals for new programs such as health and long-term elderly care begin to win broad public support.

SOCIAL FORCES: WELL-EDUCATED AND FAMILY-ORIENTED BABY BOOMERS

Other characteristics of the baby boom group affect dominant social values. This cohort is the first that is college educated on a mass basis. At least one-half of the cohort has attended college, and one-quarter of that group has completed four or more years of college. This pattern will hold for subsequent cohorts as well (see figure 3). This is a threefold increase over the generation that matured in the 1950s. The impact of a college education is hard to measure, but, over the late 1980s and early 1990s, the dominant force seems to be summed up in two words: sophistication and skepticism.

Figure 3
Educational Attainment: Percent Population with 4+ Years of College (Ages 25 to 29)

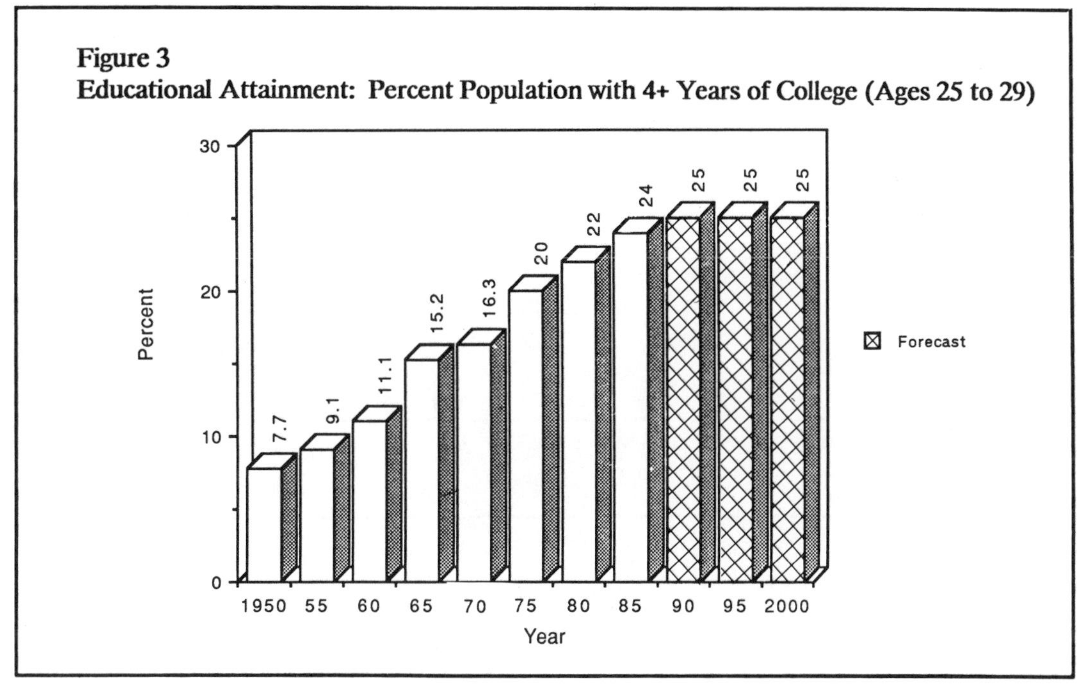

In the health care field, these two characteristics mean a more selective and careful use of the system by consumers. Many educated consumers seem to follow the trend developed in the mid-1980s that "the more you know, the more carefully you use the system." Patients will avoid major operations and invasive procedures unless they clearly hold the promise of increasing longevity and of not threatening the quality of life. This group is much more sophisticated in its use of information available on diagnosis and courses of treatment and more skeptical about provider recommendations. In essence, this better educated group views providers more as professionals instead of unchallengeable experts.

A second characteristic of the baby boom cohort is the dominant role of young families. Although fewer households with three or more children exist now than was the case during the 1950s, the number of households with at least one child under 18 is up from 25 million in 1965 to almost 40 million in 1995. This will mean that in the late 1990s over 40 percent of all households will have a child, the highest level since the mid-1970s (see figure 4).

Figure 4
Households with Children Under 18 (Percent of All Households)

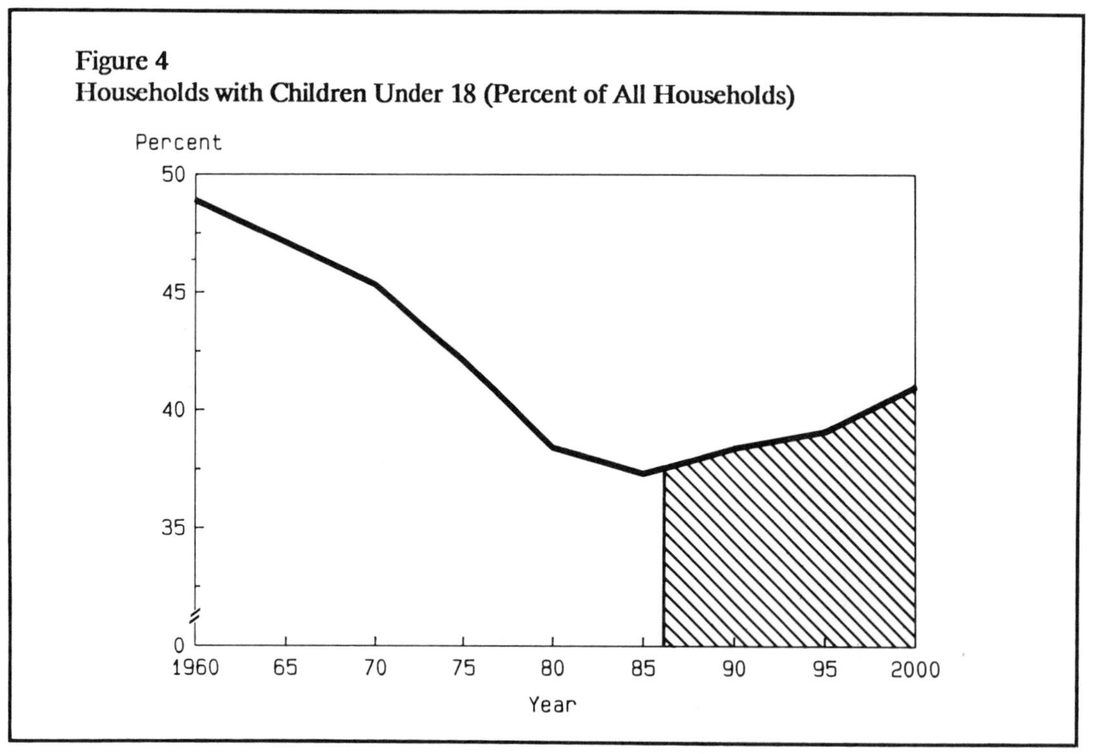

As families become fashionable again, the dominant social focus is not on health care--because young families have few high-expense health needs--but rather on housing, child care, and education. The last comparable period in the United States so dominated by young families was the 1950s, when health care spending rose only slightly faster than GNP, and public spending priorities were on local and national security, education, housing, transportation, and community infrastructure.

ECONOMIC FORCES: CONCERN OVER THE BUDGET

The economic environment moves along at a modest growth rate averaging 2.5 percent per year in real terms between 1986 and 2000. The dollar value of GNP rises from $3,998 billion in 1985 to $5,790 billion (in 1985 dollars) in 2000. This moderate growth rate reflects some key forces in operation: the slowing growth of household formation with the loss of the associated economic dynamic that new households provide; the more competitive international environment that keeps competition for the world consumer market extremely tight throughout the period; the coming of age of the baby-bust cohort, which means few new labor force entrants each year; and a less expansive government role. These factors keep overall economic growth at a lackluster rate, though well in line with the long-term real growth in the United States over the period from 1970 (see figure 5). In the meantime, inflation averages around 4 percent per year as world commodity and energy prices remain low and new labor-saving technologies and foreign competition keep new wage awards relatively modest.

Figure 5
Real GNP Growth 1985 - 2000

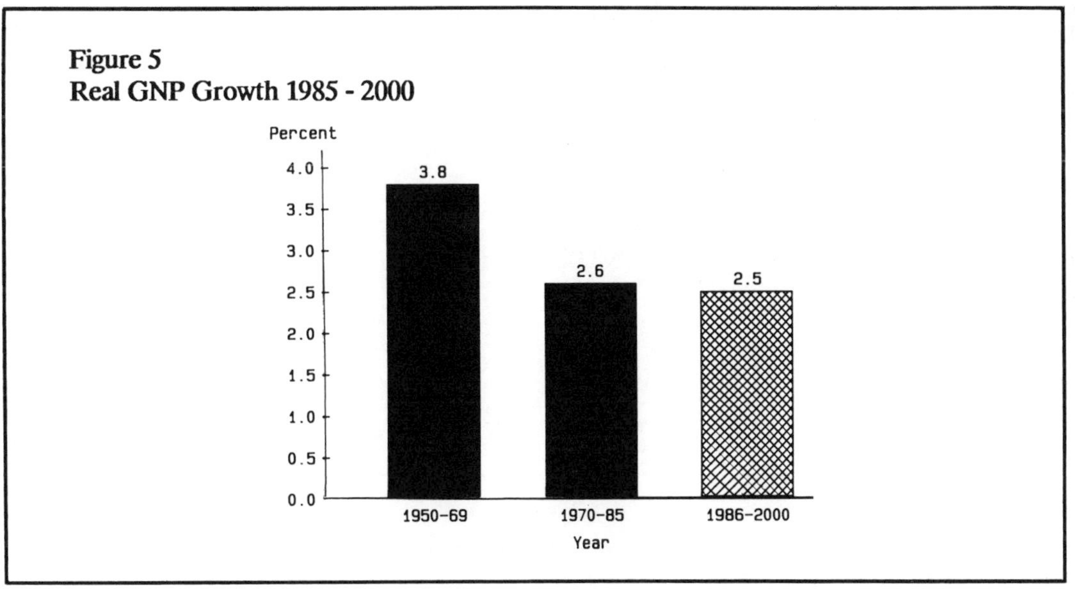

In an era of modest economic growth, the government continues to find itself in a funding crunch. The basic agenda for the government was set during the Reagan Administration when tax cuts created a sizable deficit and resistance to new taxes became an ingrained habit to householders with large personal debts. The large annual government deficits became a key constraining force on public policy choice. An outbreak of inflation in the late 1980s leads to a renewed effort to control spending and to modest tax hikes to bring the deficit under control. After reaching an average of over 3.5 percent of GNP in the mid-1980s, the total government budget deficit decreases slowly to an average of about 1.5 percent of GNP in the early 1990s and to less than 1.0 percent of GNP in the late 1990s (see figure 6). In dollar terms, the federal deficit declines to about $100 billion in the early 1990s and to about $50 billion in the mid- to late 1990s while state and local governments remain in substantial surplus. The cost of this deficit reduction is high and includes some increases in federal, state, and local taxes. However, the resistance of the baby boomers to tax increases combined with the sluggish economy ensure that tax increases are modest in size.

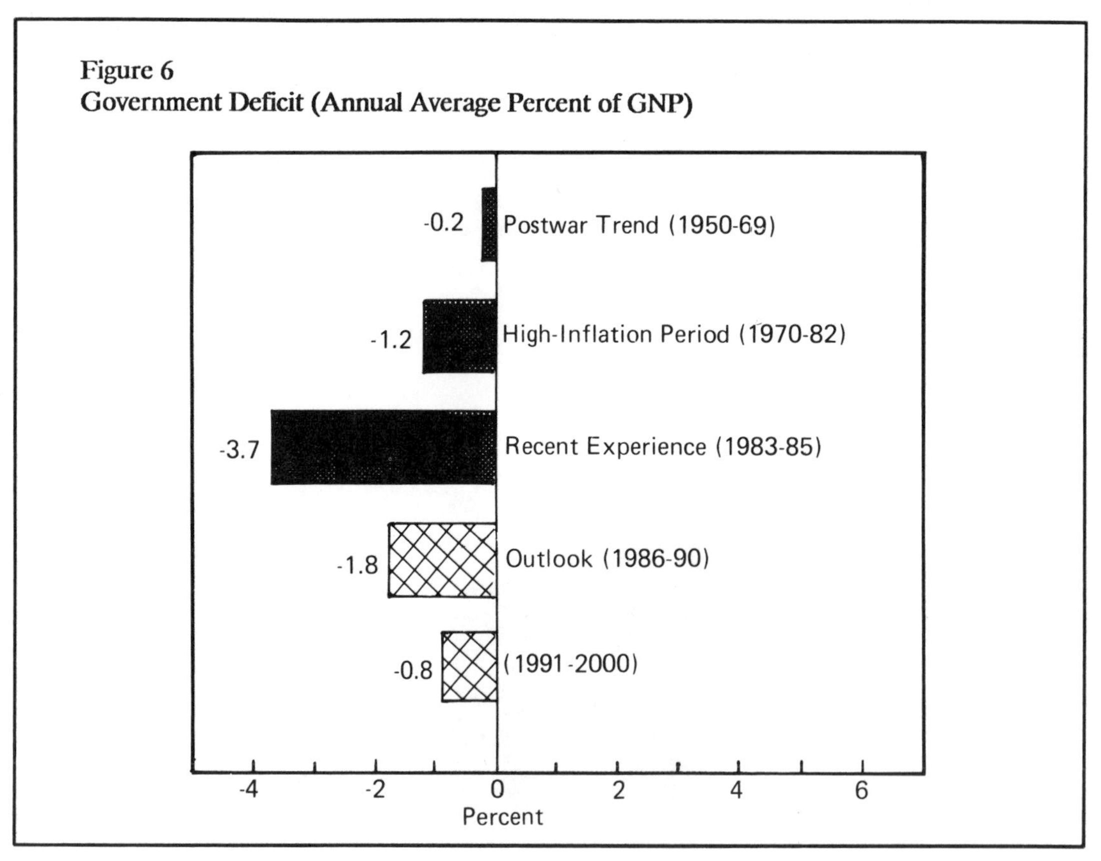

Figure 6
Government Deficit (Annual Average Percent of GNP)

Dealing with the deficit and tax resistance simultaneously has the effect of slowing the long-term trend toward an expanding role for government in society. Whereas government spending rose from 27 percent of GNP in 1960 to 35 percent in 1985, it increases to only 36 percent in 2000 (see figure 7).

Figure 7
Government Share of GNP (Percent)

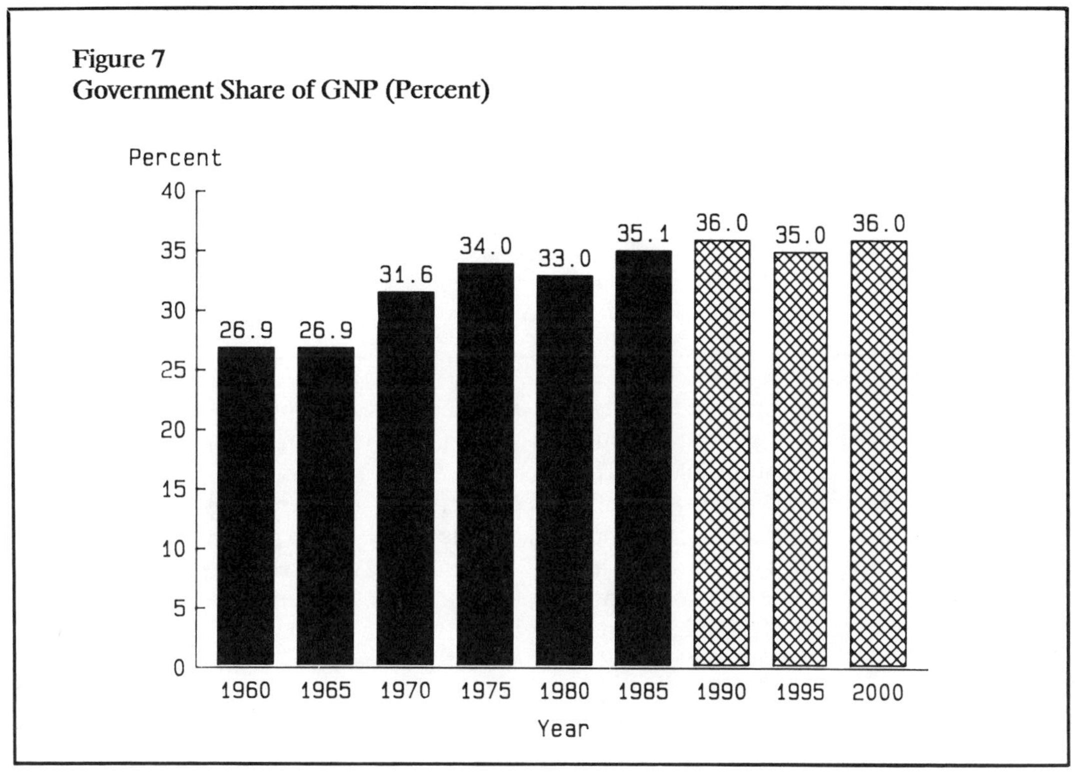

The actual dollar growth in government spending is substantial, from \$1,402 billion in 1985 to \$2,085 billion (in 1985 dollars) in 2000. Paying for the higher level of expenditures, including a narrowing of the deficit and servicing the growing national debt (which reaches \$2.8 trillion in 2000) takes some substantial increases in taxes. In the early 1990s, new tax increases are passed. Tax receipts, which accounted for 31.7 percent of GNP in 1985, increase to 34.9 percent of GNP by 2000 (see table 1).

Table 1
Government Tax Receipts

	Percent of GNP		Billions of 1985 Dollars	
	1985	2000	1985	2000
Personal taxes	12.2	**14.0**	488	**811**
Social security taxes	8.9	**9.2**	356	**532**
Corporate taxes	2.3	**3.3**	92	**191**
Indirect business taxes	8.3	**8.4**	331	**496**
Total Taxes	31.7	**34.9**	1,267	**2,020**

The increased tax burden is especially heavy on business. Corporate taxes as a percent of business profits rise from 32.7 percent in 1985 to 47.1 percent in 2000. This increased tax burden is one clear reason why business becomes adamant about controlling its own operating costs. Tax increases also hit the individual: the percent of personal income spent on direct taxes rises from 14.7 percent in 1985 to 16.9 percent in 2000. If social security payments are included, the percentage grows from 20.1 percent in 1985 to 22.4 percent in 2000.

At this point, the deficit is not the perpetual "crisis issue" that it seemed to be in the mid-1980s. Still, it remains a focus of concern and keeps the government from initiating many new or additional programs.

ECONOMIC FORCES: A COMPETITIVE CLIMATE FOR BUSINESS

For business, severe market competition remains a predominant force: competition from new technologies, competition from new market entrants and, especially, competition from foreign firms. The larger presence of foreign firms in U.S. markets is a permanent feature of the landscape. The percent of U.S. GNP spent on imports of goods and services grew from an average of 4.5 percent in the 1950s and 1960s to 8 percent in the 1970s to over 11 percent in the mid-1980s. By the mid- to late 1990s, the percent of GNP devoted to imports has grown to 14 percent, including a full spectrum of products and services that provides a competitive challenge to every major U.S. industry. When combined with the restrained economic growth rates and higher taxes, the competitive environment means that pressure on business continues. In fact, as a percent of GNP, retained business profits remain as low as they were in the 1970s and early 1980s (see table 2).

Table 2
Retained Business Profits (Average Annual Percent of GNP)

Period	Percent of GNP
1950-1969	2.9
1970-1985	2.0
1986-2000	**2.0**

ATTITUDES: CONTROL OVER THE PUBLIC PURSE AND HOUSEHOLD BUDGETS

The basic demographic, social, and economic forces already noted help mold key attitudes of the public. Attitudes are major forces in changing directions in health care. They take many years to change, and they respond to fundamental forces in our society. Thus, the momentum of change is hard to reverse. Even when problems inherent in change become prominent, it takes a long time before they work their way through to generate a response sufficient to reverse previous changes. Thus, the dominant attitudes described here have an impact on the system at least through the mid-1990s, if not longer.

The public's attitude toward government spending reflects the skepticism toward government activities that developed during the 1970s and early 1980s. A continuing perception exists that current public spending can be done more effectively, and any new program that seems to imply tax hikes meets resistance. The public seems to approve of the tax increases only if they are targeted for deficit reduction. This resistance reflects the attitudes of the dominant age group during the period of time in which traditional government services do not play a big role in people's lives. The spending priorities of this cohort are security (national defense and local police and fire) and local community-based activities (education, parks and recreation, child care, job safety, and the environment). But the dominant priority for the decade 1985-1995 is how to reduce the deficit and to maintain existing government spending constant as a share of GNP.

ATTITUDES: LESS CONFIDENCE IN MEDICINE

Public attitudes toward spending on the needs of the elderly do not undergo a major change until the late 1990s when the parents of an increasing portion of the baby boom reach old age and as the financial position of this group changes from being net debtors to that of net creditors. Then, concerns about the viability of the social security system and Medicare, as well as questions about the financing of long-term care alternatives affect the dominant perceptions of the public about the role of government and government spending.

Even then, the public continues to be careful in its choice of health care services. Because of budget pressures on government and competitive pressures on most businesses, any increase in medical costs is shared directly with the ultimate consumer. The general level of education and the availability of more information on treatment outcomes make the consumer a much more careful buyer. Business and government provide users with a wealth of information. Knowing more about the variation in medical opinions (and the inherent dangers or side effects in many procedures), an increasing number of consumers are now more skeptical about accepting the advice of those physicians who advocate complex and expensive treatment. This change in perception is best measured by public attitudes toward leaders of social institutions. Throughout the 1960s and 1970s, the public held doctors in a unique position, expressing a great deal more confidence in them than in the other most prestigious professionals--educators, the military, clergymen, and justices of the Supreme Court. By the early 1990s, the gap in confidence closes, and doctors are seen by the general public as no different than these other professionals (see figure 8).

Figure 8
Public Confidence in Leaders of Institutions
(Percent Expressing "A Great Deal of Confidence in . . .")

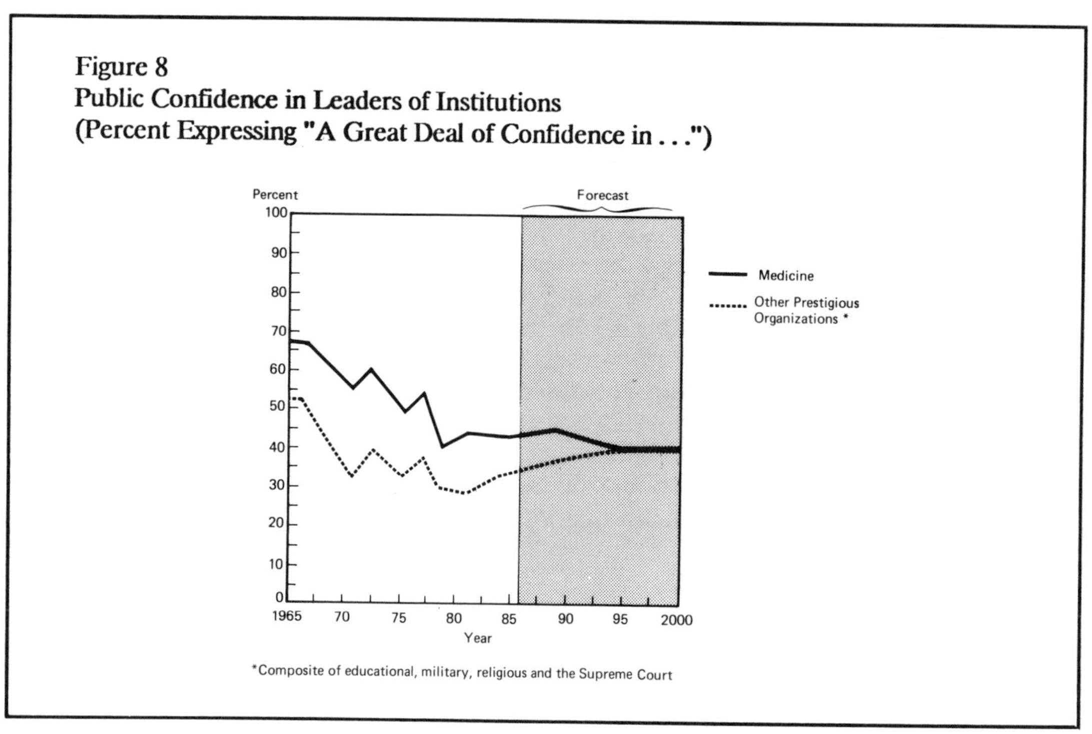

*Composite of educational, military, religious and the Supreme Court

Another change in attitude is important as well--the attitude about the right of people to refuse the use of extreme and costly measures to prolong life. Again, better information is essential in changing attitudes toward extreme cases: information about costs to the system and the relationship between prolongation and the quality of life. In addition, a consensus builds in many cases in which patient, family, doctor, and clergyman agree that the individual has a right to refuse heroic measures to prolong life. As table 3 shows, the attitudes toward those favoring individual and family choice of the right-to-die when faced with "incurable diseases" have been shifting markedly. Medical practice adapts to these changed attitudes in many communities, focusing on early detection, prevention, and functional remedies in both research and care rather than heroic measures in the last days of life.

Table 3
People Favoring the Right-to-Die for Those with Incurable Diseases
(Percent of All Poll Respondents)

Year	Percent
1973	37
1977	49
1981	56
1985	61
1990	**72**
1995	**82**
2000	**85**

Setting Relative Priorities

PUBLIC POLICY AND HEALTH CARE

The most severe constraints on government policy are primarily budgetary. Virtually all funds raised by tax increases in the 1980s and 1990s are applied to reduce the budget deficit. This means that the government's expenditures as a share of GNP rise very slowly through the period 1986-2000. Competition for shares of that government spending is intense. The relative priorities for spending are determined by the concerns of the baby boom cohort, and their concerns are those of mid-life: education, community safety, the poor, and the environment. A series of national polls taken in the mid-1980s confirmed this set of relative priorities, and these priorities held through the early 1990s (see figure 9). It was a long enough period, though, to have a profound impact on patterns of government spending.

Figure 9
Public Spending: Public Priorities
(Percent of Public Who Feel That We Spend "Too Little on . . .")

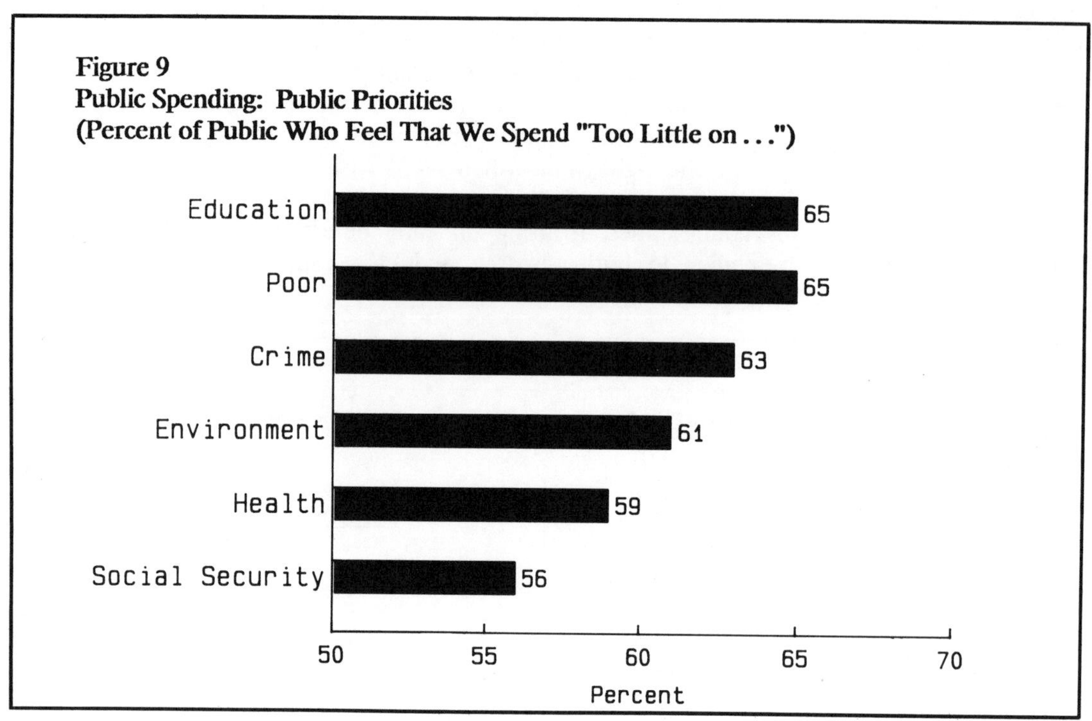

Public opinion priorities translate into spending priorities. Table 4 outlines the distribution of all government spending over the period 1960-2000. The share of defense spending declines slightly after its rise in the early 1980s, but the long-sought "defense dividend" never appears because a new generation of defense systems and the cost of maintaining a stable conventional force with a shrinking number of 18-year-olds requires a sizable allocation of budget funds each year. As the children of the baby boom cohort reach school age, elementary and secondary schools experience an enrollment increase of from 10 percent to 15 percent, and baby boom parents set a top priority on money for school expenditures. Concerns about the aging, the homeless, and the disabled keep spending on social insurance and welfare payments high. Other budget spending increases reflect the baby boomers demand for local services--police, court, fire, and recreation; the nation's demand to be economically competitive--national R&D, resource and energy research, the space program, and retraining; and environmental concerns--waste disposal and cleanup, infrastructure rebuilding. Continuing high interest payments--the fruit of the large deficits of the 1980s--continue to take a relatively large portion of the budget.

Table 4
Government Spending (Percent of All Spending)

	1960	1970	1980	1985	**2000**
Defense	32.6	23.4	15.1	18.5	**17.9**
Education	13.7	17.9	17.0	15.0	**16.6**
Social insurance/welfare	16.5	19.2	26.0	22.0	**21.8**
Health	4.4	8.8	12.1	12.9	**12.8**
Other social	5.1	4.1	4.1	2.8	**3.0**
Interest	5.6	4.8	5.8	9.9	**9.1**
All other	22.1	21.8	19.9	18.9	**18.8**
	100.0	100.0	100.0	100.0	**100.0**

All in all, given national priorities, the ability of health care expenditures to hold their own as a share of total government spending indicates a strong political influence. In constant dollar terms, government spending on health rises on average 2.7 percent per year, from $181.5 billion in 1985 to $267 billion in 2000.

The government also is extremely active in containing health care costs, through the use of its regulatory and legal powers. Some universal care programs, like Medicare, are subject to higher levels of copayment. Diagnosis Related Group (DRG) rules are extended to certain types of physician services, and various other fixed price reimbursement rules are tried at both the federal and state levels. Through its reimbursement rules, the government fosters the establishment of preferred providers that specialize in Medicare, Medicaid, and other government-paid programs. In fact, in some states medical school loans are tied to a period of service in such publicly oriented provider organizations. Finally, many state governments make substantial changes in the rules for torts: caps are put on liability claims for pain and suffering and on lawyers' contingency fees; some bellwether states eliminate the legal notion of joint and several liability, which makes any party who contributes to an injury through negligence potentially responsible for the entire injury award.

Another public policy benefit that flows from the more constrained environment in health care is the smaller inflationary impact of health care price increases on overall inflation rates. Over the fifteen years from 1961 to 1985, medical care costs rose almost 30 percent faster than other costs (during the last five years of that period, they rose 60 percent faster). During the fifteen years from 1986 to 2000, medical care costs, responding to a more competitive marketplace and institutional cost control measures, rise on average only slightly faster than the overall CPI.

BUSINESS AND HEALTH CARE

The business community became extremely concerned about health care in the early 1980s. Over the previous decade, employers from medium and large companies offered group health insurance to their employees because of legal requirements and employee benefit considerations. Because of tax benefits and inflation, the full cost impact of these benefits was either not too noticeable or was easily passed on to the consumer.

The situation changed dramatically in the early 1980s. Inflation rates plummeted, making it more difficult to pass through cost increases. Foreign competitors entered the relatively open and expanding U.S. market in droves. And deregulation and new technologies brought new competitive forces to many U.S. markets. Many U.S. firms experienced an increase in competition and a narrowing of profit margins. In this context, the sharp rise in the cost of health care benefits became apparent to all corporate managers. Between 1970 and 1985, health care costs more than doubled as a percent of total compensation (see figure 10).

Figure 10
Burden of Health Care Costs on Business
(Health Care Costs as a Share of Total Compensation)

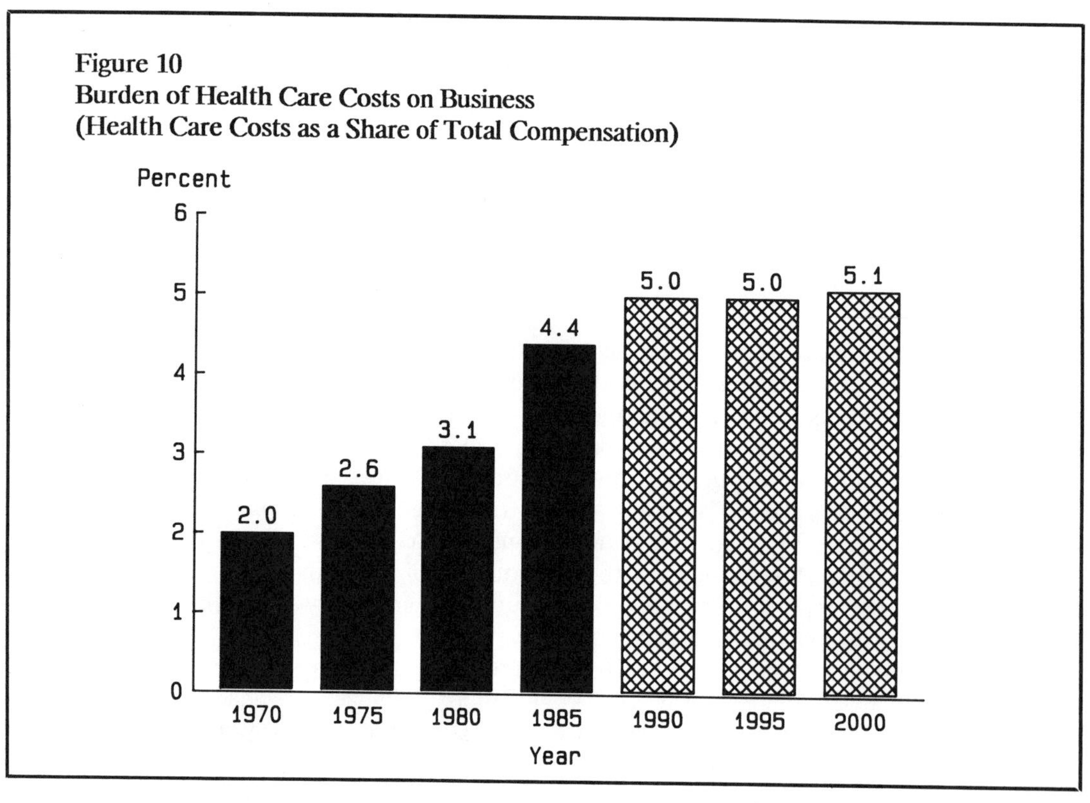

During the late 1980s, such benefits become an obvious target of cost control programs. The business response is to work closely to support institutional innovations that provide cost control opportunities, to involve business in monitoring providers, and to pass on a share of the costs to employees. Cost savings get wide support in the business community because every dollar saved in health benefits has a direct bottom line impact on total compensation and eventually on corporate profits.

Corporate benefit managers exert substantial pressure on insurers to become their agents for cost-effective service. The enhanced power of information technologies allows managers to monitor employee health care use patterns and to monitor both community use patterns and the relative performance of some innovative community health care groups. Government databases on health care performance undergoes a major transformation through the increasing application of more sophisticated recordkeeping and analysis of health care statistics. Insurers work with businesses to tailor programs to take advantage of these improved sources of information. Because of the much more aggressive cost-containment policy, the share of compensation going to health care levels off during the early 1990s.

SOURCES OF HEALTH CARE FUNDS

The attempt by each of the major payers to control the impact of escalating health care costs leads to some sharp conflicts: the business sector tries to control compensation costs by increasing copayments; individuals concerned about rising out-of-pocket costs demand more coverage from public and employer benefit programs but resist more copayments and taxes; and the government, facing huge budget deficits, passes legislation mandating employers to extend employee coverage. The effort at "passing the buck" is not successful, but it does lead to consensus of support for structural reforms that promote constraint.

The shares of payments made by some of the key payers shift modestly. Government's share increases slightly during the period from 1985 to 2000, but this increase is wholly a demographic phenomenon, reflecting the 22 percent increase in the number of individuals 65 and over whose use of the health care system is intense. It also reflects the recognition that certain key problems such as the elderly, the uninsured, and those hit by health-related catastrophes are the responsibility of the government (see table 5). The increased consumer share (and the smaller business share) is an attempt to revise the incentive structure of the system to increase copayments by the middle class user. This is a conscious attempt to increase individual responsibility for paying for a portion of care--putting some direct economic incentives into each patient care decision. After twenty years of sharp decline in share, consumers react to the increased burden by being more careful in their use of the system, adding an awareness of cost to their existing concerns over quality and access. Private philanthropy, which used to account for a substantial flow of funds for constructing and equipping community hospitals, finds a much diminished role in the restructuring of the 1990s.

Table 5
National Health Expenditures: Sources of Funds

Shares Paid by:	1985		2000	
	Billions of 1985 Dollars	Percent	Billions of 1985 Dollars	Percent
Government (all level)	175	41.1	**266**	**42.8**
Business*	123	29.0	**175**	**28.0**
Consumers**	116	27.2	**175**	**28.0**
Private (other)	11	2.7	**6**	**1.0**
	425	100.0	**622**	**100.0**

*Includes only employer contributions to group health insurance.

**Includes consumer direct payments (out of pocket) and health insurance purchased by the consumer.

Structural Change

NEW INCENTIVES

The context fosters two related driving forces: the growing concern of payers over cost and the need of providers to identify and capture new markets. These forces are sufficient to change the structure of the health care delivery system during the 1980s and early 1990s. The first driving force--the rising cost of health care services and the growing responses of the key payers--was evident from the early 1980s. Each of the payers tries several distinct lines of action. The government's response is to impose DRGs, restrict cost-of-living increases on reimbursements, and raise copayments on Medicare. Business, on the other hand, pushes up copayments, makes use of alternative delivery systems, and imposes requirements for second opinions. Individuals begin to do more shopping around for insurance plans and providers.

Such payer actions stimulate limited structural adjustments. A number of new organizations emerge to offer what they say are more cost-effective health care services: for-profit hospitals, HMOs, IPAs, and PPOs. The decline of public confidence in medicine spurs such experimentation. But it proves harder than expected to redistribute the type of care provided in a well-entrenched sector in which consumer trust plays a more important role than economics. By the mid-1980s, only about one person in five in the private care market is covered by contract or capitated care services.

A second force, however, comes into play in the mid- and late 1980s: the emerging problems of providers finding customers. From the 1960s to the 1980s, the expanding health care market attracted new resources--talented young people who spent eight to ten years in training to become physicians--and new hospital beds; the expectation was that such resources would be needed ten years in the future. The market changes in the mid-1980s bring quite an abrupt shift in the outlook for physicians and hospitals.

Hospital admissions fall dramatically from a high of 36.4 million in 1981 to 33.5 million in 1985. Length-of-stay drops as well, from 7.6 days to 7.1 days, decreasing total patient days from 278.4 million in 1981 to 238 million in 1985. Hospital administrators face a growing problem of how to fill beds or how to develop new community services that could offset the fall in the number of inpatients. At the same time, the inexorable growth in the number of new doctors continues apace. Between 1976 and 1985, the annual number of MD graduates doubled (from 8,300 in 1976 to 16,300 in 1985). This influx of new practitioners makes it extremely difficult for young physicians to start a practice. By the mid-1980s, 40 percent of post resident MDs entering practice are accepting salaried positions.

Institutional managers--whether they be for-profit corporate directors, hospital administrators, insurance company managers, or physicians who direct or administer group practices--are quick to take advantage of these market opportunities. They establish a new role as intermediaries between the payers who are concerned about cost and the providers who are concerned about markets. Traditionally, in the 1960s and 1970s this intermediary role was merely that of a broker--usually in the form of third-party insurance--that passed on the costs of the providers to payers in the form of annual rate increases in premiums. By the 1990s, these managers are taking a much more active role in organizing the system. Through direct salaries or contracts, they organize the providers, particularly those who have trouble gaining a market position by themselves or those who have special services or expertise that can be used in a wider market to provide integrated services for a given payer group.

Figure 11 highlights the major change that takes place in the health care system between the 1970s and the 1990s: the emergence of a major role for health care managers who organize providers and compete aggressively for markets. These managers are more willing to accept a constrained reimbursement environment because they have more control over the organization and delivery of health care services and are more effective in controlling cost pass-throughs.

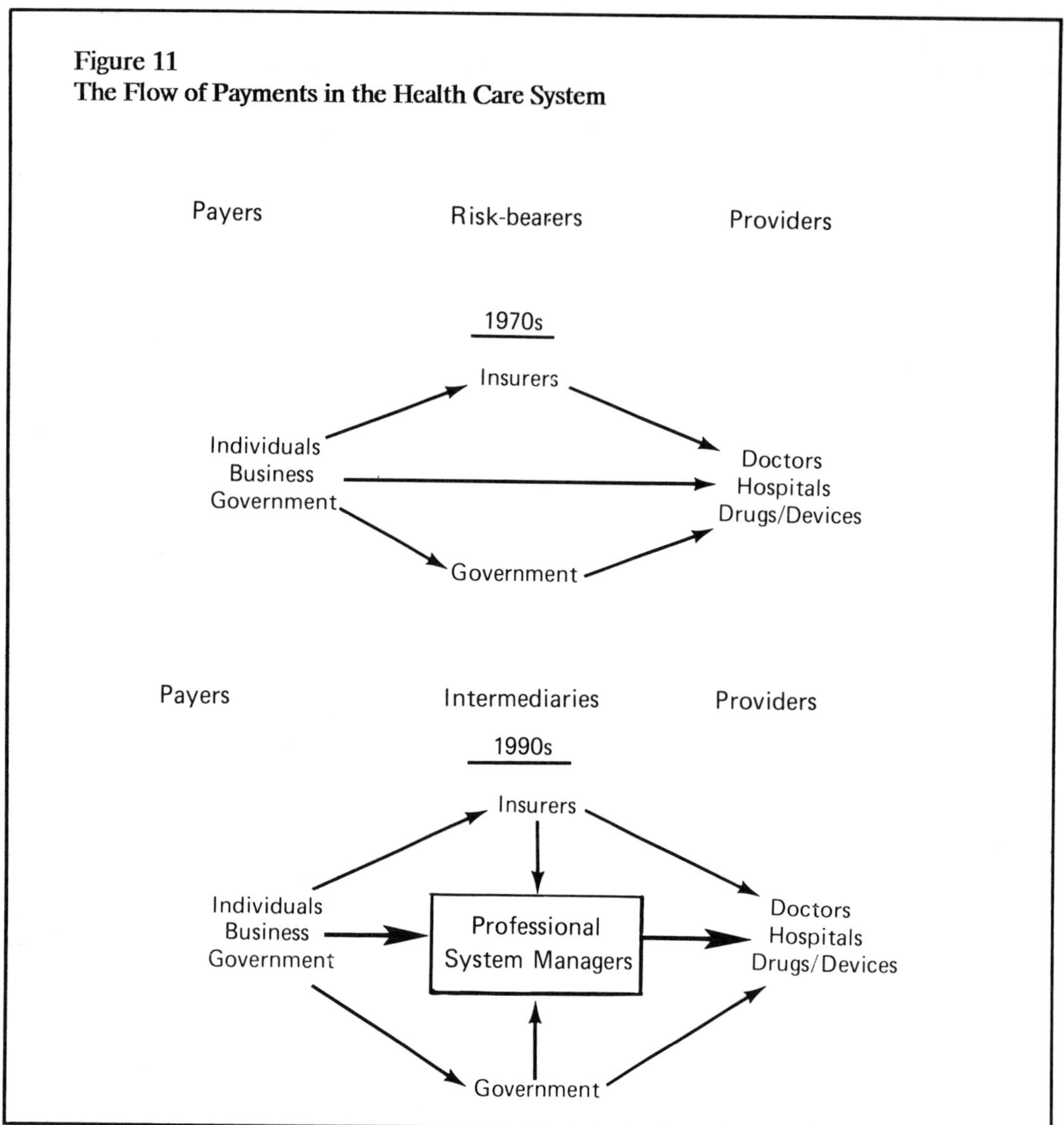

Figure 11
The Flow of Payments in the Health Care System

THE TRANSFORMED SYSTEM

The frenzied activity to find alternative system structures among insurers, providers, and government that was so prominent in the mid-1980s finally shakes out in the 1990s to reveal some clear transformations. Table 6 shows a sharp drop in the portion of the population covered in fee-for-service arrangements between 1985 and 2000 with compensating increases in those covered under contract or capitated plans. There is little change in the portion who are outside of the system (those who do not use the health care system at all or who receive uncompensated care). The major shifts involve a fall in the share of the population covered under strict fee-for-service systems, even when such systems include substantial copayments or employer review programs (such measures as utilization review and mandatory second opinions).

Table 6
The Changing Structure of U.S. Health Care (Percent of Total Population)

	1975	1985	2000
Out of System:	10	10*	9**
No care	5	5	5
Uncompensated care	5	5	4
Fee-for-Service (FFS):	87	72	40
Comprehensive	15	5	5
With copayment only	67	28	15
FFS with copayment and review	5	39	20
Contract:	1	8	23
Selective contracts and review	--	3	20
Fixed contracts per episode	1	5	3
Capitated:	2	10	28
Plans with individual practitioners	--	6	18
Plans with a single group	1	3	8
Full service integrated facility	1	1	2

*Assumes that 15% of the total population is uninsured, of which 5% gets care on a FFS basis.

**Assumes that 12% of the total population is uninsured, of which 3% gets care on a FFS basis.

In general, employer review programs are useful as a means of gathering information on employee use patterns and the effectiveness of specific types of programs. Eventually, such information leads to more enduring contractual arrangements with either independent providers or groups of providers. The contracts span a wide range of institutional settings, from controlled fee-for-service contracts with individual physicians through capitated plans with integrated providers. The range indicates that many individuals or families can preserve some degree of choice as to health care coverage. Still, the large number of people enrolled in some form of capitated payment system (almost 30 percent of the total population) is the driving force that establishes reimbursement limits for the contract care sector and the fee-for-service sector. Within the capitated payments sector, the most successful players in enrolling customers are not the fully integrated HMO-types of providers but capitated plans negotiated with a series of providers (both physician groups and hospitals). These plans allow some patient choice among groups of physicians and hospitals but force all of the enrolled physicians and hospitals to provide a high level of cost-efficient care as determined by the prime contractor (either business/government or an agent such as an insurer acting on their behalf).

The system is not foolproof: many payers do not have the resources to assure both cost effectiveness and quality; the bureaucratic controls are cumbersome and inefficient; practice changes or new technologies are difficult to track within the system without strict rules on utilization which often slow innovation; and access problems affect some within the insured care system as well as those with no insurance coverage. Still, the system has made major strides in bringing a sense of cost efficiency into the day-to-day operation of the health care system.

The structural changes have some major impacts on the relative positions of various actors (see table 7). In sum, physicians' share of the spending pie decreases and a much larger portion of their income is earned in the form of salaries or as members of group practices where clinical and economic autonomy are restricted. Hospitals' share of total spending goes up modestly. A portion of that spending results from the greater intensiveness of inpatient care, but most of the increase reflects the growth in revenues from outpatient activities--clinics, ambulatory care units, imaging centers, surgicenters, blood banks, regional labs, and alternate care centers--sponsored and/or managed by the hospitals. The share going to nursing homes rises sharply as the number of the very old goes up. The administrative cost of managing the system increases. A portion of this administrative cost is picked up as an increase in spending on insurance, although both hospitals and doctors gain a substantial part of the "management" fees within the system. There are winners and losers among the academic medical centers as well. The premier institutions continue to attract research funds, and their hospitals find a role as "first class" providers. The second tier group develops a much stronger service orientation, often at the expense of its academic functions.

Table 7
Relative Shares of Health Care Spending

	1985		2000	
	Billions of 1985 Dollars	Percent	Billions of 1985 Dollars	Percent
Physician Services:				
Self-employed	82.8	19.5	83.0	13.3
Salaried/managed	10.3	2.4	22.4	3.6
Hospitals:				
Inpatient	131.4	30.9	171.6	27.6
Outpatient	25.0	5.9	73.5	11.8
Nursing Homes	35.2	8.3	60.0	9.7
Insurance: Administration and profit	26.2	6.2	45.0	7.2
Other	114.1	26.8	166.5	26.8
	425.0	100.0	622.0	100.0

Into the 21st Century

The newly structured system still offers a broad range of choice to most Americans, and it does not lack technological sophistication--indeed, it is widely thought that the system uses technology more effectively than it ever did. Further, the flow of resources into the system reflects society's trade-offs with other critical public needs. In the late 1990s, pressures begin to build for reform to meet the needs of an aging society. The baby boomers are now confronting the problems of aging parents; they are realizing their own mortality and reflecting on the burden this will place on their children. The health care agenda begins to change from concern about building an efficient system to concern about financing the huge burden of the baby boomers as they age. A summary of the environmental and overall health care system changes occurring in Scenario I (and contrasted with Scenario II) appears in Appendix F.

Scenario II: Health and Wealth

Overview

The historic pattern of growth in the health care system continues in the 1990s, despite best efforts at cost containment. The rate of growth is somewhat slower than in boom periods such as the 1970s, but the trend toward increasing expenditure on health care as a share of GNP is clearly upward--following the temporary, relatively shallow dip during the cost containment years of the mid-1980s. This upward trend is driven by demographic, attitudinal, technological, and political forces and sustained by economic developments. These forces create pressures to provide a wider range of health care services to an aging and technologically sophisticated population. On balance, such pressures are stronger than the countervailing forces favoring fiscal conservatism; consequently, health care expenditures rise through 11 percent of GNP in the late 1980s to 12 percent in the early 1990s, and reach 12.7 percent by the end of the century (see Figure 12). This translates into health care spending of $790 billion in 2000, an 80 percent increase over 1985 levels. While GNP will grow at an average rate of 3 percent annually, total spending on health care will rise by 4.2 percent per year. This complex system keeps on developing because people want more health care, and the institutions exist to provide it.

Figure 12
U.S. Health Care Spending (As a Percent of GNP)

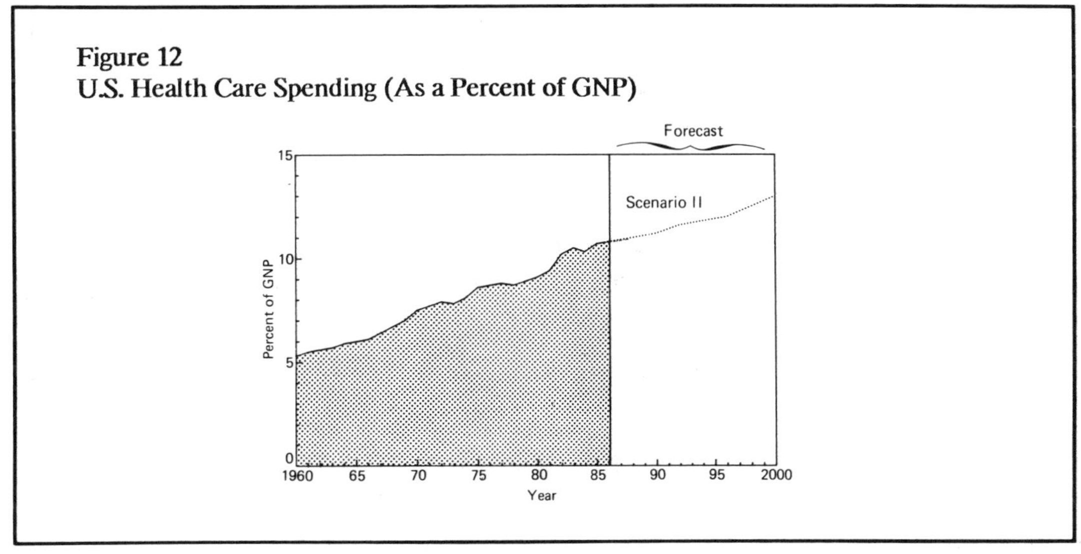

Forces for Growth

ATTITUDES: PEOPLE WANT MORE

The attitudes toward health care can be summed up as "more, but not more of the same." Although individuals continue to regard their own physicians in relatively high esteem, respect for the system declines steadily through the late 1980s. By 1987, it becomes clear that the health care system is not delivering the full range of services that people (particularly the elderly) want, and increasingly the public favors improving access to the system for the uninsured. Consumers are interested in new forms of services and new locations of care that improve the convenience of the system and that fill the service gaps in traditional medical care. For example, consumers in the mid-1980s make it clear to providers that what they need is: extended hours of operation for health facilities; more home health care; adult day care facilities; nursing homes; wellness programs; drug and alcohol treatment and rehabilitation; and improved transportation services. But these perceived needs are in addition to, rather than at the expense of, traditional acute care services.

A second key attitude that plays an important role in driving the system is acceptance of medical technology. The attitudes that began to build in the late 1970s and 1980s--a questioning of medical technology in general and of heroic medicine in particular--are prevalent in the 1990s with regard to care for the terminally ill. However, demonstrable progress has been made in the early diagnosis and more successful treatment of a wide variety of diseases: breast and colon cancers, some mental illnesses, and coronary artery disease are notable examples. This progress has not produced cures, but the benefits of the treatments are measurable and well publicized. People accept that these interventions are worthwhile, and pressures build to make them available. (Baby boomers are particularly conscious of the progress in breast cancer and coronary artery disease--illnesses that they are beginning to encounter among their age cohort. The elderly, on the other hand, are particularly attracted to those interventions aimed at debilitating illnesses such as Alzheimer's.) The United States places great store on science and technology in the 1990s; consequently, support for and confidence in the generation and application of scientific knowledge increases (see figure 13) as does the use and sophistication of medical technology in the hospital, the doctor's office, and the home.

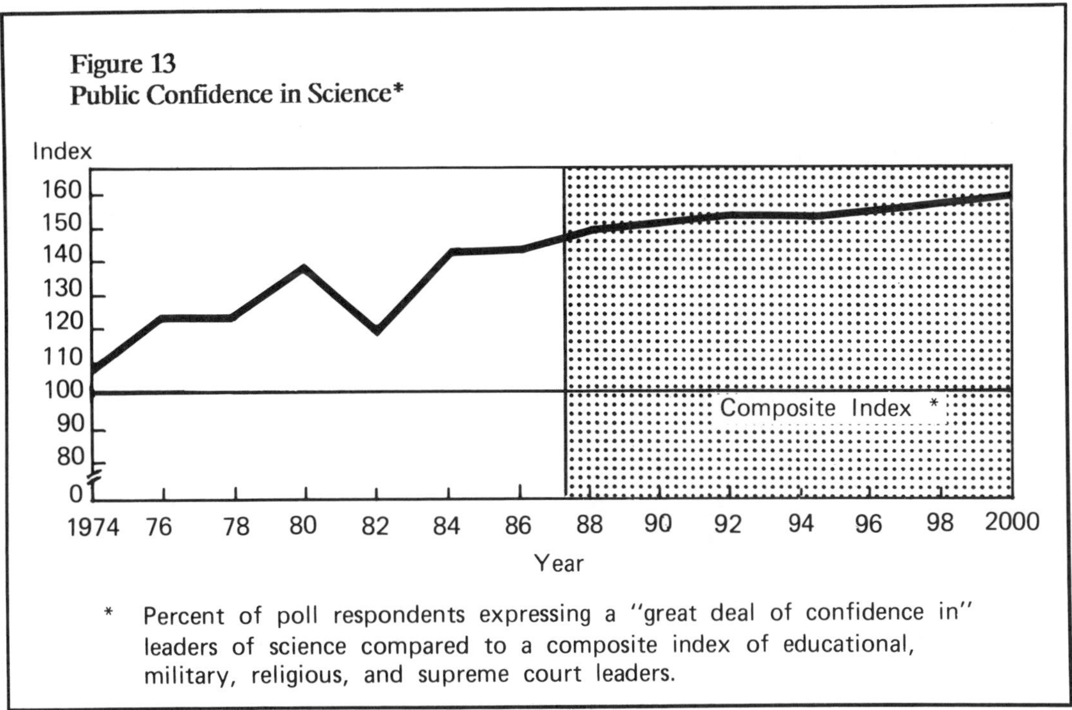

The net result of these prevailing attitudes is widespread public support for expanding the range of chronic, acute care, and rehabilitation services; and for increasing the sophistication and diffusion of medical technology. Somewhat paradoxically, the hospice movement continues to grow because in many illnesses the limits of medical science are obvious to the public. In such circumstances, patients and their families are electing social support systems rather than heroic medical intervention.

DEMOGRAPHICS: THE AGING OF AMERICA

A key factor governing the growing demand for health care lies in the aging of the U.S. population. As the population ages, attitudes change, and each cohort produces different pressures on the health care system. The number of people over 65 increases from 28.5 million in 1985 to 35 million in 2000. The elderly continue to place a disproportionate weight on the health care system: because of the natural incidence of morbidity in this group and its demand for an increased range of services, and because of its increasing political clout in shaping health policy. But the increasing number of elderly is really comprised of three different groups (see figure 14). Each group has its special demands: the "young old" (65-75) demand acute care services and rehabilitation; the "old" (75-85) demand not only their share of acute care services but also long term care, home care, and rehabilitation; and the large expansion of the "very old" (over 85) creates special demands for custodial care.

Figure 14
The Growing Number of Elderly (Millions)

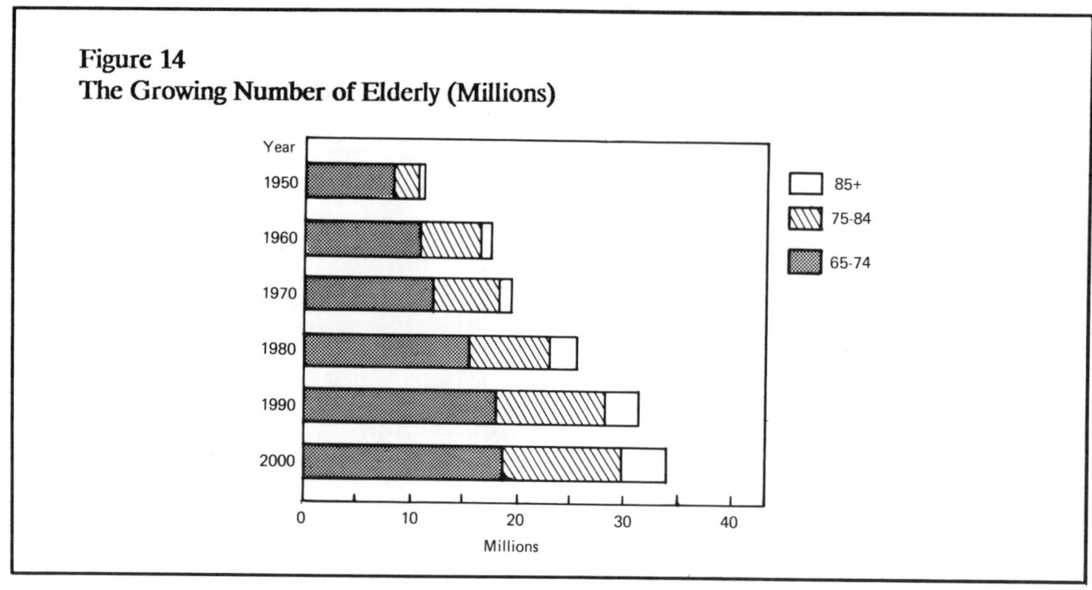

The elderly are not simply an extrapolation of past generations of "old people." They are qualitatively as well as quantitatively different. For example, the elderly of the late 1990s have education levels that more closely resemble those of the rest of the population (see figure 15), making them more consumerist, and they spearhead the reaction to many cost containment practices that they find objectionable.

Figure 15
Education Gap Narrows (Median Years of Education by Age)

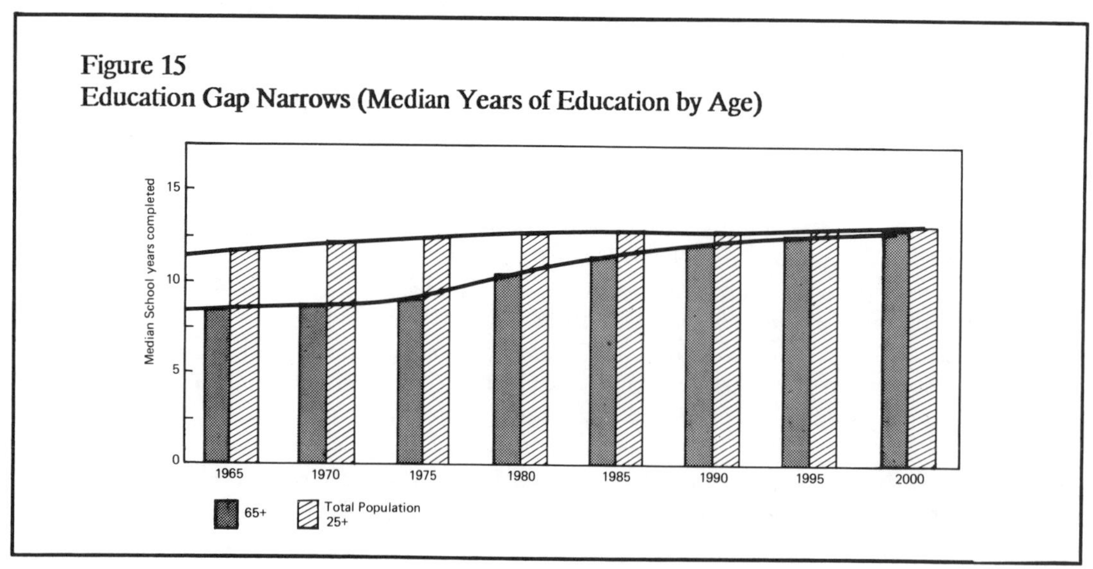

The "no-care zone"--the no man's land between posthospital discharge and self-sufficiency with chronic disability--is particularly worrisome to the elderly and their families who are unable or unwilling to shoulder these care burdens as part of regular "household chores." For example, in the period from 1985 until 2000, disability days among the elderly increase by 31 percent. About 80 percent of care for the frail elderly is provided by their families, principally daughters. Yet, as working baby boom women age into their fifties, they simply have no time and no financial incentive to provide that care. Figure 16 shows the increased proportion of workers among middle-aged women over this period.

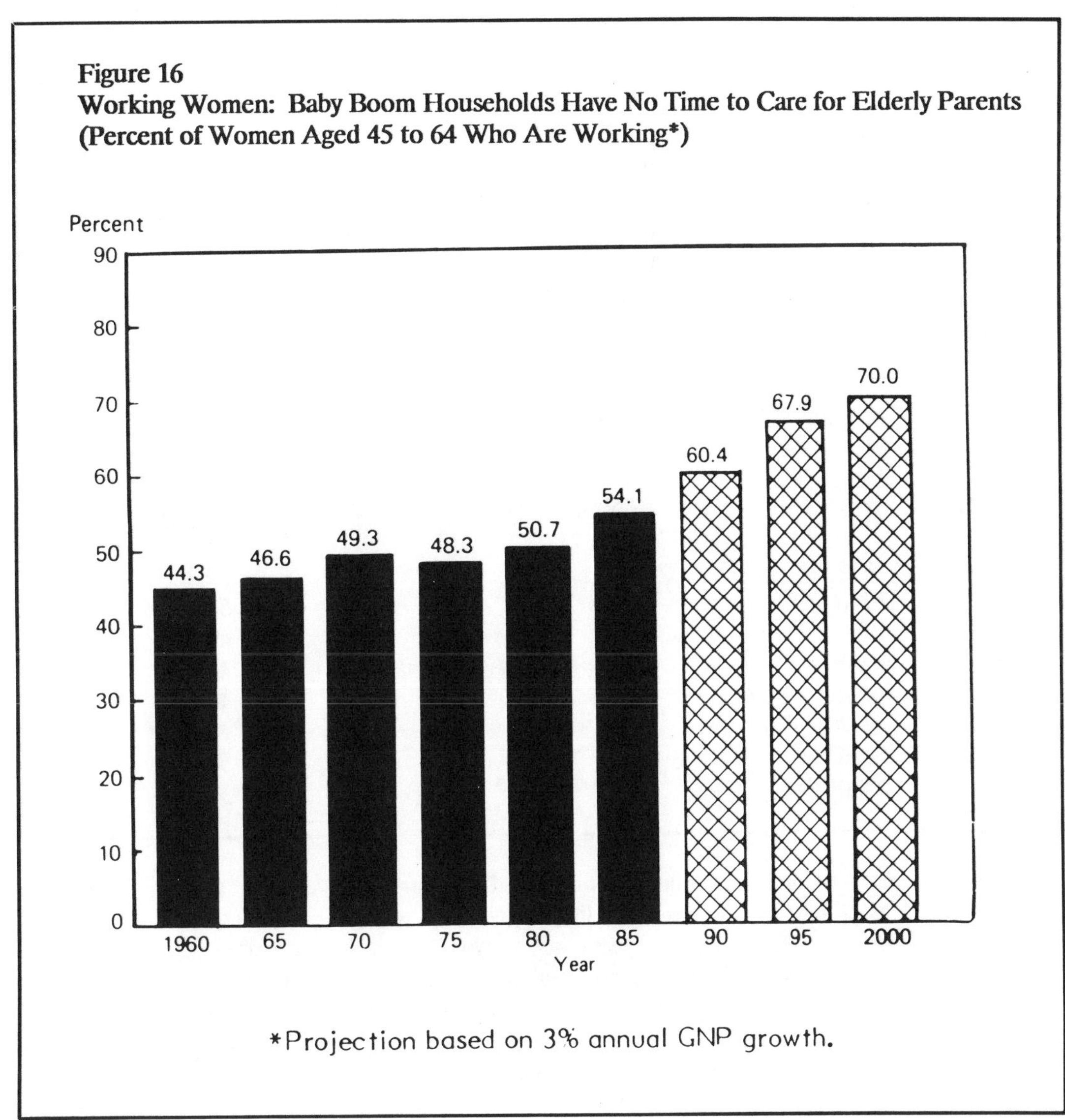

Figure 16
Working Women: Baby Boom Households Have No Time to Care for Elderly Parents (Percent of Women Aged 45 to 64 Who Are Working*)

*Projection based on 3% annual GNP growth.

It is a common belief that DRGs are the prime cause of the "no-care zone," and attitudes favor spending money to correct the situation. A priority is placed on posthospital rehabilitation, long-term care, and home support facilities, but this often comes in addition to, and not at the expense of, acute care services. This is because the elderly are not alone in demanding better care. Technological advances and steady growth in personal incomes increase the demand for care among all age groups, making it impossible simply to shift resources between cohorts.

Similarly, the aging of the population creates interesting political coalitions. The large group of the population over 45 is politically important because it represents both the elderly *and* their large cohort of children, the baby boom. In combination, they have a strong interest in the quality and availability of health services.

The over-45 group is a strong political force in the 1990 congressional elections and stronger still in 1992 (see table 8). As a majority of voters, the elderly and their concerned middle-aged children bring health care once again to the forefront of the national agenda, spearheaded by groups such as the American Association of Retired Persons (AARP) that continue to gather momentum. Thus, the perceived inadequacies of the health system become a key policy issue in the late 1980s and early 1990s.

Table 8
Voters in Presidential Elections by Age (Percent of Voters)

Year	Young (18-44)	Middle-Aged and Old (45+)
1972	50.2	49.8
1976	49.9	50.1
1980	50.5	49.5
1984	51.9	48.1
1988	**51.6**	**48.4**
1992	**50.6**	**49.4**
1996	**49.0**	**51.0**
2000	**45.9**	**54.1**

Aging is a phenomenon of the labor force as well as the population as a whole. Increases in life expectancy at age 65 mean that the elderly have at least twenty years of active life to be constructively filled (and paid for), and these more educated elderly tend to keep working longer in their white-collar jobs than blue-collar employees did in the past.

An older work force means higher health care costs for business, particularly those firms in old, heavily unionized industries. Retiree benefits also are a major liability for these firms, which keeps business involved in the care of former workers. Equally important for business at the other end of the labor force is the paucity of new labor market entrants, which makes benefit packages a tax efficient way to attract and retain talent. Business, however, does not completely forget the lessons from the cost containment years. Firms continue to monitor and critique health care delivery, and they impose certain management controls on the providers of health services for their employees. Overall utilization and access to health care, however, are being driven by the needs and wants of an aging and technologically sophisticated set of consumers.

TECHNOLOGY: THE PROMISE OF PROGRESS

Technology is not driving the health care system, but technological progress is giving increasing legitimacy to the health care enterprise. The late 1980s prove to be a turning point in the development of a wide range of technologies. Biotechnology has provided new tools for diagnosis, treatment, and research. Such mechanisms help push the dispersion of diagnostic testing to the doctor's office and to the home, a shift motivated by the financial incentives of the DRG era. At the same time, there has been a range of developments in "halfway technology"--those technologies that create some benefit but do not cure. Progress in immunology, genetics, and bioengineering has produced a range of expensive but relatively effective diagnostic and therapeutic systems. For example, progress in the management of immunosuppressed patients (brought about largely by extensive basic and applied research on AIDS) has given new tools to both physicians and surgeons. Those tools improve the outcome of organ transplantation and make it an even more popular procedure. Cancer therapy becomes increasingly sophisticated, and steady but not revolutionary progress is made as a result. The biggest improvements in health outcomes are gained when early diagnosis is coupled with these sophisticated interventions. Successes are well publicized in the *New England Journal of Medicine* and the *National Enquirer* alike, adding to high public demand for access to these technologies.

Cancer is not the only area in which early diagnosis and more sophisticated therapies make some gains. Coronary artery disease can be diagnosed earlier using a combination of imaging and genetic diagnostic studies and treated in many cases using genetically engineered drugs. Alzheimer's is readily diagnosed using MRI technology, and some progress is being made in the management of these patients using sophisticated drug therapy. Further, developments in fertility diagnosis and therapy, as well as microsurgery and neonatal care, are opening a whole range of possibilities in enhancing reproduction and sustaining low-birth weight infants. However, all of these technologies are ameliorative rather than curative--they are expensive substitutes for effective prevention or cure. As such, they vastly increase the costs of care.

Widespread diffusion of all of these promising technologies is not immediate. In the late 1980s, diffusion of "halfway technologies" is impaired by the lingering obstacles of cost containment; these constraints diminish greatly by the late 1990s. Certain technologies are proved to be cost effective, and their diffusion is encouraged, perhaps overencouraged. As with the early days of x-rays, many patients get unnecessary treatments. These patterns are legitimized by the gains in quality care that medical technology makes possible in the 1990s.

PUBLIC POLICY: PRESSURES AND CHOICES

The 1992 election consolidates the shift away from cost containment. A number of factors influence the shift. The political weight and leverage of the elderly grow steadily through the late 1980s and early 1990s (see table 9). The DRG system, which was supposed to be the cornerstone of cost containment for the federal government and for many states and private insurers, proves to be too complex, too unwieldy, and too unpopular to hold its ground as a cost containment tool. Business has been affected by the increasingly tight labor market--employees want more flexibility in their benefit packages, and they are willing to supplement health benefits out of pocket in order to get the right "package" for their own family needs. Business also feels increasing pressure to expand retiree benefits. Hospitals are complaining that they have been unfairly discriminated against because Medicare did not succeed in applying a DRG-like scheme to physicians; consequently, hospitals have carried the burden of cost containment. Finally, the states and the federal government are getting increasing political flak on the problems of the uninsured and underinsured. The time is right for change.

Table 9
Top Ten Swing States in Presidential Elections

State*	Electoral College Reps 1984	Percent of Population Over Age 65 1984	1990	2000
NY	36	12.7	13.6	13.9
TX	29	9.5	10.1	9.9
PA	25	14.1	15.7	16.3
OH	23	11.9	13.1	13.9
FL	21	17.6	20.3	21.5
MA	13	13.4	14.4	14.7
NC	13	11.2	12.9	14.4
GA	12	9.9	11.1	11.8
MO	11	13.6	14.2	14.3
WI	11	12.8	12.8	12.9
	194 (36%)			
U.S. average		11.9	12.8	13.1
Number of states above U.S. average		6	8	7

*States were selected based on a history of party change in outcome over four presidential elections (1972, 1976, 1980, 1984), then ranked according to electoral college representation. They represent 36% of the electoral college votes.

Governments--both federal and state--have tried to patch up the cracks in the health care system in the late 1980s. But their piecemeal efforts are seen as inadequate. The real problem is that people are not getting what they want: access to high quality health care at reasonable personal cost. If it takes more of their tax money to achieve this, then that is what must be done.

Health care is never very far away from the top of the national political agenda. In the late 1980s, however, health care's claim on national resources is more rigorously examined than in previous decades. The reason, of course, is the federal deficit, which remains the intractable legacy of the Reagan years. Despite the popularity of tax cuts, it becomes painfully apparent to political leaders in the late 1980s and early 1990s that the government deficit is not a spending crisis but a revenue crisis. The political fallout of draconian spending cuts is far greater than that from an incremental increase in the taxation of affluent middle class Americans. "Revenue enhancement" enables government spending as a share of the economy to creep up to 38 percent of GNP, up from 35 percent in 1985 (see figure 17) or, in 1985 dollar terms, an increase from $1.4 trillion to $2.4 trillion.

Figure 17
Government Share of GNP (Percent)

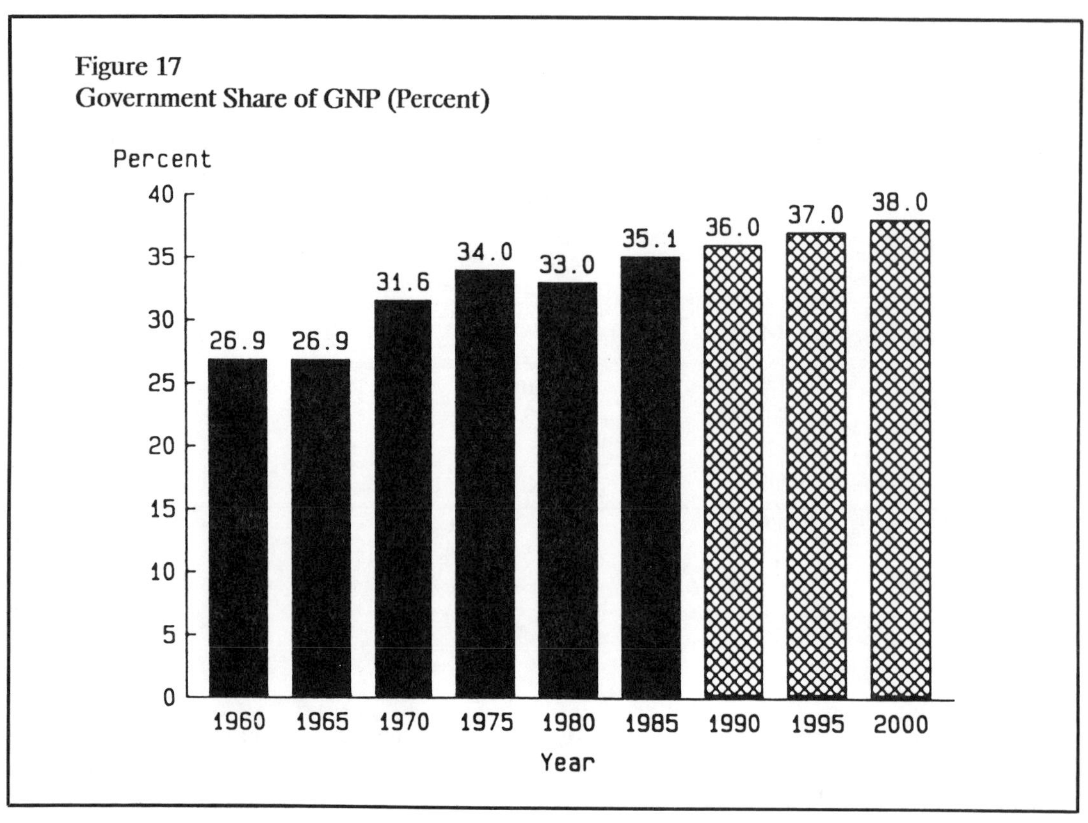

The increase in government spending is not evenly distributed among the competing claims. Table 10 shows that two areas--education and health--are given relatively higher priority than defense or other social programs. These two areas have demographic drivers. For government health expenditures, it is the aging of the population over 65 years of age. For education, it is the movement of echo boom children through elementary school in the late 1980s, through high school in the 1990s, and into the college system by the end of the century.

Table 10
Government Spending (Percent of All Spending)

	1960	1970	1980	1985	2000
Defense	32.6	23.4	15.1	18.5	**15.5**
Education	13.7	17.9	17.0	15.0	**15.5**
Social insurance/ welfare	16.5	19.2	26.0	22.0	**22.2**
Health	4.4	8.8	12.1	12.9	**14.0**
Other social	5.1	4.1	4.1	2.8	**2.8**
Interest	5.6	4.8	5.8	9.9	**11.0**
All other	22.1	21.8	19.9	18.9	**19.0**
	100.0	100.0	100.0	100.0	**100.0**

These relative shifts in priority do not imply reductions in other programs. Table 11 shows that all sectors (except for defense) grow at least as fast as the economy as a whole. As the U.S. continues to consume services at an increasing rate relative to goods, government expenditures (predominantly service oriented) involve a larger share of the economy.

Table 11
Government Spending

	1985		2000		
	Billions of Constant 1985 Dollars	Percent of All Spending	Billions of Constant 1985 Dollars	Percent of All Spending	Average Annual Growth Rate 1985-2000 (Percent)
Defense	259	18.5	**367**	**15.5**	2.4
Education	210	15.0	**367**	**15.5**	3.8
Social insurance/ welfare	308	22.0	**525**	**22.2**	3.6
Health	182	12.9	**332**	**14.0**	4.1
Other social	39	2.8	**66**	**2.8**	3.6
Interest	139	9.9	**260**	**11.0**	4.3
All other	265	18.9	**450**	**19.0**	3.6
	1,402	100.0	**2,367**	**100.0**	3.6

But the differences in growth rates are important and reflect the soul searching about priorities of the post-Reagan era. The public views social spending on many specific programs as absolutely necessary, and the political pressures against cuts prove too difficult to resist.

Although expansion of health care receives strong public support, the government faces a real policy dilemma in designing specific programs. The president is elected in 1988 on the basis of moderate to liberal social values and, at the same time, fiscal conservativeness. Promises to review Medicare have to be kept, but the administration is being told by Health Care Financing Administration (HCFA) planners that any reform in the late 1980s and early 1990s has to be robust enough to weather the coming fiscal crisis of 2010 when the first of the baby boom hits 65. The response for Medicare is in the form of a slightly higher deductible for those who can afford it, coupled to catastrophic insurance. The government also regulates posthospital discharge care standards, provides tax incentives for long-term and rehabilitation care insurance and puts pressure on businesses to expand benefits for their retirees. Some states elect in their Medicaid program to follow the federal government's lead; others continue with their own versions--particularly those eastern states where a system of cross-subsidization has been developed between the insured and the uninsured. Overall, however, the rising tide of sentiment in support of improving services and expanding access for the working uninsured loosens the funding constraints on government.

These measures gain broad support for three principal reasons. First, the elderly have spearheaded the reforms using key swing states in the Northeast and the Middle West as their political base (see table 9). Second, the baby boomers are not prepared for a reemergence of the extended family as a means of social support, and they are willing and able to pay taxes to ensure that the new nuclear family is not threatened by their aging parents and grandparents. They also are mindful of the upcoming inevitable decline in their own health status and are eager to make sure some kind of umbrella system is in place. Third, the support comes because people believe that progress in technology will eventually make this system work. While not quite there, cost-effective medical technologies seem to be just around the corner.

ECONOMY: DOING WELL ENOUGH

These expansions in health care spending are sustained by the performance of the economy: governments, households, and businesses are not as economically constrained as in the previous period of health care reform in the early 1980s. Moderate to strong growth through the mid-1980s dips into an inevitable but shallow recession in the late 1980s, which aggravates the negative effects of DRGs and adds to the pressures for Medicare and Medicaid reform. Growth then rebounds strongly through the 1990s. Overall real economic growth from 1986 to 2000 averages a moderately healthy 3 percent (see figure 18), resulting in a real GNP of $6,230 billion (1985 dollars) by the year 2000.

Figure 18
Real GNP Growth, 1950-2000

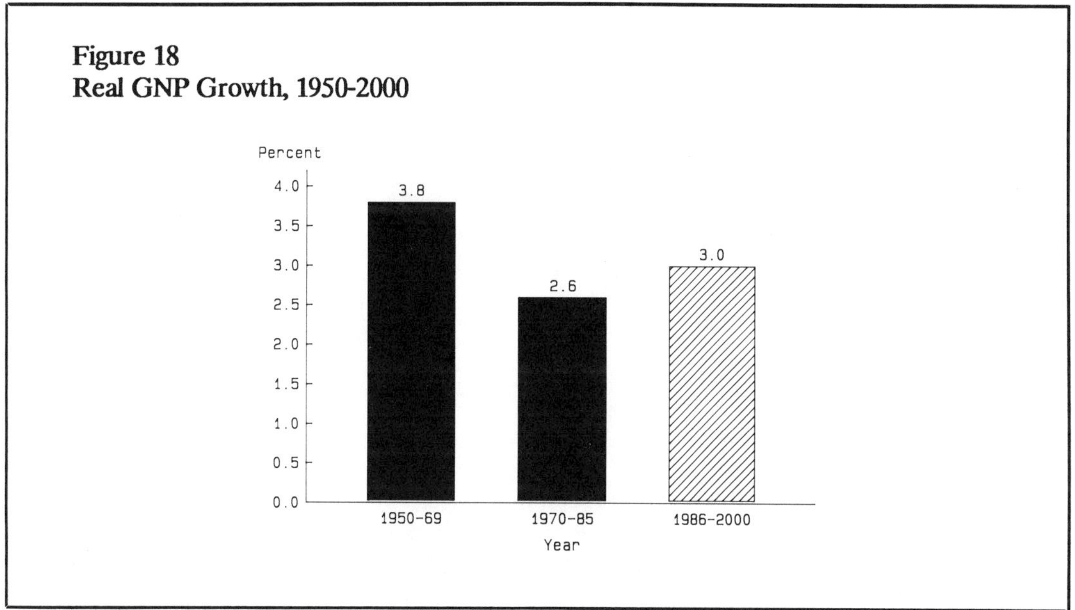

This growth creates real gains in income for business, government, and households. The really important economic factor for health policy, however, is the way in which a combination of steady economic growth, low inflation, an improving balance of trade, and higher revenues has allowed the U.S. government to ameliorate the budget deficit problem. By the mid-1990s, a deficit still exists, but it is perceived as manageable. And, just as inflation did in the 1980s, the deficit moves down the policy agenda. Although Americans continue to favor fiscal conservatism, there is agreement that government can afford certain programs where the political will is strong enough. This flexibility is increased by the relative cuts in defense spending as superpowers begin to recognize that arms escalation is just too expensive.

Business has done reasonably well. It has raised productivity steadily by successfully applying new technology to old industries, and it has faced foreign competition by improving the organization and quality of domestic production.

But, although business is doing better in a growing economy, retained business profits do not keep pace for three key reasons. Competition is still severe domestically and internationally, and many once high-profit businesses are brought into the competitive fold: telecommunications and electric utilities are notable examples. Second, inflation is eroding profit rates--in particular for service industries--as labor costs rise. Third, taxation levels are very much higher than was the case in the mid-1980s (see table 12).

Table 12
The Tax Burden (Percent)

Year	Consumers Tax as a Share of Personal Income*	Business Tax as a Share of Business Profits**
1960	12.6	47.7
1965	12.1	38.7
1970	14.3	48.2
1975	13.5	46.1
1980	15.7	48.3
1985	14.7	32.7
2000	**16.9**	**49.9**

*Excludes consumer contributions to social insurance.

**Corporate profits with inventory valuation adjustments and capital consumption adjustments.

Higher levels of taxation help close the deficit gap by the end of the century, but the national debt of $2.36 trillion still has to be serviced (which accounts for the 11 percent of government expenditures going to interest at prevailing rates that are fluctuating between 9 percent and 11 percent). The expansion of spending and the deficit reduction have been achieved at great cost to American taxpayers (see table 13). But mainstream American households and businesses are doing well enough to afford it. In comparison to most other industrialized nations, real incomes are higher and tax rates are lower. Consequently, little resistance is felt to the gradual creep upward in taxation in general and spending on health care in particular. Society as a whole views health care as a superior good: an increasingly affluent nation will consume more of it.

Table 13
Government Tax Receipts

	Percent of GNP		Billions of 1985 Dollars	
	1985	2000	1985	2000
Personal taxes	12.2	**15.0**	488	**934**
Social security taxes	8.9	**11.0**	356	**623**
Corporate taxes	2.3	**3.5**	92	**218**
Indirect business taxes	8.3	**8.5**	331	**529**
Total Taxes	31.7	**38.0**	1,267	**2,367**

Sources of Health Care Funding

The growth in the economy has a major effect on the health care spending patterns of the various actors. Government gives way somewhat more than business does (see table 14). All levels of government come out of the Reagan years with a lower revenue base and a lower share of spending on social programs. As discussed earlier, through the 1990s, this situation gradually reverses itself, taxes are raised, and social spending by government creeps back up as a reflection of specific political pressures and changing public priorities (see table 15). In particular, this growth in the government share reflects the increase in spending for the over-65 population and the inclusion of the uninsured and underinsured (particularly AIDS patients) in state and federal health programs. Health expenditures for these groups, although supported by premiums from consumers, flow through government channels.

Table 14
National Health Expenditures: Sources of Funds

	1985		2000	
	Billions of 1985 Dollars	Percent of All Spending	Billions of 1985 Dollars	Percent of All Spending
Government (all levels)	175	41.1	332	42.0
Business*	123	29.0	224	28.4
Consumers**	116	27.2	215	27.2
Private(other)	11	2.7	19	2.4
Total	425	100.0	790	100.0

*Includes only employer contributions to group health insurance.

**Includes consumer direct payments (out of pocket) and health insurance purchased by the consumer.

Table 15
Government Percent Spending (All Levels)

	1975	1985	2000
Government spending as a share of GNP	36.2	34.5	38.0
Social spending as a share of all government spending	57.4	52.7	54.5
Government health care spending as a share of all social spending	18.0	23.0	25.7

The net result of these shifts in emphasis is that government's bill for health care almost doubles in real dollar terms from $175 billion in 1985 to $332 billion in 2000 (see table 16).

Table 16
National Health Care Expenditures: Sources of Funds (Billions of 1985 Dollars)

	1985	2000	Net Increase 1985-2000
Government	175	332	157
Business	123	224	101
Consumers	116	215	99
Private (other)	11	19	8
Total	425	790	365

But the other payers do not escape the inflation in costs. Business increases its real spending on health care by $101 billion (over 80 percent in real terms). This involves an increase in the share of total employee compensation going to health care premiums from 4.4 percent in 1985 to 5.4 percent in 2000 (see figure 19), a figure that belies the enormous increase in taxes on business (see table 12), some of which end up in government health spending.

Figure 19
Burden of Health Care Costs on Business
(Health Care Costs as a Percent of Corporate Compensation)

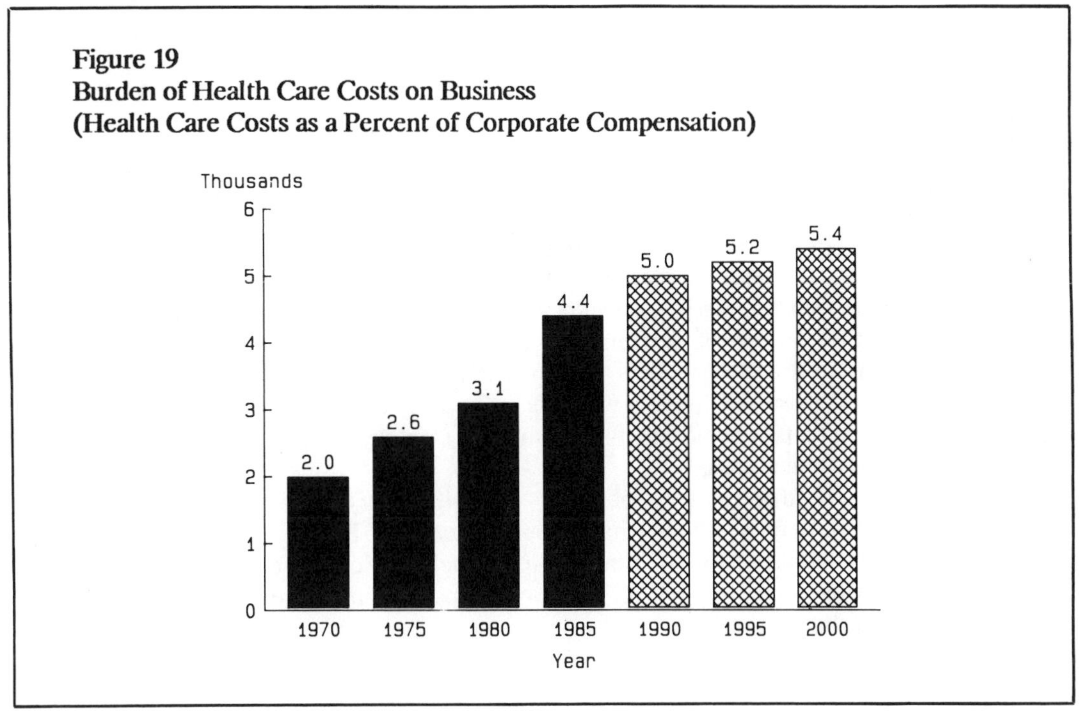

Similarly, on the consumer side, expenditures almost double, which reflects two important but somewhat inconsistent effects by two distinct tiers of the populace. First, a group of unwilling consumers is shouldering the burden of higher deductibles and copayments. Although direct health care costs are still a very small component of consumer expenditures (approximately 5.3 percent, up from 4.1 percent in 1984), certain groups--particularly elderly women living alone--are still paying over 10 percent of household expenditures on health care (see table 17). Even with the expansion in catastrophic coverage for Medicare and the new initiatives for the uninsured in the late 1980s, inflation in health care costs and the continued existence of copayments and deductibles keep the "barriers to entry" relatively high for certain groups.

Table 17
Consumer Expenditures on Health Care
(Percent of Total Expenditures by Urban Consumer Units)

Age of Reference Person	1984	2000
Under 25	2.3	2.4
25-34	2.9	3.0
35-44	2.9	3.5
45-54	3.7	4.5
55-64	4.6	5.2
65-74	8.4	8.0
75+	13.3	12.0
Total (all consumer units)	4.1	5.3

In contrast, a second group of consumers (who used to be called YUPS in the 1980s but who by the late 1990s are dubbed MARFs--middle aged rich families) are willingly spending more out of pocket. This group is the darling of health care marketers. They are purchasing long-term care insurance products for themselves and their aging parents; they are enrolled in self-funded wellness programs; they buy the services of health consultants of various types; and they actively support home-based health care technologies.

A final category of payers (private other) is comprised of the philanthropic organizations that support health. Prudent management and a favorable investment climate keep their endowments relatively high, and they continue to actively seek out gaps and pressure points in the system that they can remedy.

Structural Change

The demands of an aging, affluent, and technologically sophisticated society, when coupled with an innovative health care system, create powerful pressures for expansion. On balance, such pressures are stronger than the countervailing forces favoring fiscal conservatism. Health care is a superior good: a more affluent society spends more on it. Consequently, health care expenditures rise through 11 percent of GNP in the late 1980s to 12 percent in the early 1990s, and reach 13 percent by the end of the century. This translates into health care spending of $790 billion in 2000 (in 1985 dollars), an 80 percent increase over 1985 levels. While real GNP grows at an average rate of 3 percent annually, total spending on health care rises by 4.2 percent per year. This complex system keeps on developing because people want more health care and the institutions exist to provide it.

The most salient feature of the health care system in the 1990s is simply the enormous amount of money being spent. Spending nearly doubles in real dollars, from $425 billion in 1985 to $790 billion in the year 2000; from $1,771 per person to $2,950. But this growth comes from new services and programs, added on to, rather than substituting for, previous medical practices. There is a marked increase in the range and volume of new services such as preventive care, custodial and rehabilitative geriatric care, vision care, drug and alcohol treatment, mental health services, home services, and high-technology care such as organ transplantation. Table 18 shows the changes in health care spending taking place over the 1985-2000 period.

In the mid-1980s, cost containment pressures spurred organizational realignment and management innovation. The system does not reach a steady state. Instead, an increasingly wide and complex array of financing and delivery arrangements continues to emerge in the 1990s. These experiments are not all aimed at cost reduction; rather, they are aimed at capturing payers and patients. Diminished incentives for permanent structures limit the rigid vertical integration of providers and insurers, and businesses are less inclined to involve themselves directly in employee health care. Instead, the shakeout of the early 1990s brings marketing securely into health care, and the system becomes characterized by a plethora of new products, specialized markets and niches, decentralization of service, and an increase in consumer sovereignty.

Table 18
Total Health Care Spending: National Health Accounts (Billions of 1985 Dollars)

	1985	2000
Services and Supplies:		
Hospital care*	156.4	288.0
Physicians' services*	93.1	162.0
Dentists' services	27.1	32.0
Other professionals	12.6	36.0
Drugs, sundries	28.5	52.0
Spectacles, appliances	7.5	20.0
Nursing home, elder support	35.2	92.0
Other	11.0	12.0
Subtotal: personal care	371.4	694.0
Administration, profit	26.2	49.0
Public health	11.9	17.0
R&D and Construction:		
Noncommercial research	7.4	13.0
Construction	8.1	17.0
Total	425.0	790.0

*Physicians' services in hospitals are included in physicians services, not in hospitals, as they are in the National Health Accounts.

HYBRID HEALTH CARE

After a brief fling with vertical integration of insurers and providers, the health care industry again separates the two functions. Rigid vertical integration of insurers owning and controlling providers, or of provider ownership of captive insurers, no longer seems to work when the incentive structure deemphasizes cost containment and increasingly emphasizes capturing market share. Instead, providers integrate horizontally, seeking capital for expansion, access to managerial skills, and links to providers with complementary products that will appeal to different health care consumers. With their access to equity capital, for-profit providers again begin to expand market share after the retrenchment of the mid-1980s.

In this environment, the insurer's role as payment processor is transformed into one of performance monitor, service packager, program marketer, and information broker. The use of flexible benefits programs in the insurance industry parallels the continued innovation on the provider side. The result is a system of hybrids. Hybrid plans are offered increasingly by employers. They started in the 1980s as triple options--an HMO, a PPO, and traditional indemnity insurance--but, by the 1990s, employee benefits have become a complex smorgasbord of life, health, disability, pension, and even auto insurance. Employees are tailoring packages to suit their family needs and using elements within the packages for different purposes. The two-job household has an especially rich set of choices: his dental, her medical, his life, her pension.

Within these flexible benefits packages, employees have a wide and somewhat confusing array of health benefit options. A January 1989 *Wall Street Journal* article, "Employee Health Benefits: The New Synonyms," describes three types of plans that industry analysts argue are identical in cost for employers, in access for consumers, and in flexibility and income for providers. The three plans are:

1. An insurance company's indemnity product that incorporates administrative controls on employees' access and providers' behavior as well as an incentive bonus for physicians who keep total fees per patient below preset targets.

2. An offering from one of the aggressive Blues called a Select Health Network that allows employees access to a range of providers---those that agreed to be on-line to the insurers for billing, utilization review, and referral control purposes. Patients also pay some deductibles.

3. An offering by a new physician-owned joint venture that calls itself a Health *Management* Organization. It offers access to a range of member physicians and participating hospitals on a prepaid capitated basis, but also offers "cash back" discounts to employees for minimizing their visits to providers.

The boundaries become so blurred that no one talks about HMOs and PPOs anymore. In fact, most consumers and employers don't even know or care what the theoretical structure of the plan is; they focus more on the quality and value of the services provided.

Providers, too, have become flexible. Very few hospitals or physicians derive their patients from one source. Individual doctors and hospitals continue to sign up with a variety of intermediaries as a means of hedging their bets and accessing new streams of patients. But the system doesn't settle down as everyone expected. Instead, consumers--both individual patients and the employee benefits managers--are presented with a richer set of choices each year.

In this new world, the incentives to restrict the use of services are not stringently applied (most providers quickly become "preferred," and the differentiation among providers comes more from product mix and quality characteristics). Generally, the patients and providers of the 1990s see very little difference between plans based on fee-for-service insurance with managed care components and those that operate on a contract or capitated basis. Capitated plans continue to grow in popularity, but the enrollees perceive them as providing better value (wider range of covered services), not just cheaper health care (see table 19).

Several shifts in emphasis underlie the changes in the structure of the health care system during the 1990s: more stress on the choices made by the ultimate consumer, the rapid growth in types of services provided, and a withdrawal by government and business from the micromanagement of health care.

Table 19
Structure of U.S. Health Care (Percent of Population)

	1975	1985	1990	1995	2000
Out of the System:	**10**	**10***	**9**	**7**	**4****
No care	5	5	4	3	2
Uncompensated	5	5	5	4	2
Fee-for-Service:	**87**	**72**	**66**	**64**	**63**
Comprehensive	15	5	4	5	5
With copayment only	67	28	18	12	10
With copayment and review	5	39	44	47	48
Contract:	**1**	**8**	**13**	**15**	**17**
Selective contracts and review	--	3	6	8	9
Fixed contracts per episode	1	5	7	7	8
Capitated:	**2**	**10**	**12**	**14**	**16**
Plans with individual practitioner	--	6	8	10	12
Plans with a single group	1	3	3	3	3
Full service integrated facilities	1	1	1	1	1

*Assumes that 15% of the total population is uninsured, of which 5% gets care on a FFS basis.

**Assumes that 6% of the total population is uninsured, of which 2% gets care on a FFS basis.

AN INCREASE IN CONSUMER SOVEREIGNTY

The growth in market power of the consumer results from the increased dollars that they have to spend. Economic growth raises disposable income; at the same time, changes in reimbursement systems in the 1980s increase deductibles and copayments for all forms of public and private insurance. With more of the total bill coming out of their pockets, consumers demand the right to choose how their health care dollars are spent. This is true for both employer- and government-sponsored health plans of the 1990s.

The 1990s health care consumers also are more educated in general, and specifically about medical issues. While not believing that health care is a commodity like soap, they still insist on getting cost effective quality care, with the emphasis on quality. The cost containment period had only a temporary impact on medical spending, but it did scar the collective consumer psyche with the fear of low quality care. Although no consensus exists about how to measure quality, many people are willing to pay extra for the amenities and "hotel functions" that they associate with good care, as well as for access to the best and most recent technologies. This demand for quality, however defined, translates into a willingness to pay more for care in the hope of ensuring a better outcome, or at least a more civilized and humane experience. Consumers value the freedom of choice of providers--both physicians and hospitals--and they tend to make those judgments based on local knowledge and word of mouth more than on national advertising campaigns for multi-unit systems. In addition, consumers insist on access to procedures and technologies they have heard about in the media, and refuse to condone social policies that would limit their distribution through rationing. Finally, the growth in numbers and incomes of consumers, particularly among the elderly, increases the demand for health care and the clout that patients have with the government and providers.

GROWTH OF NEW PRODUCTS AND MARKET SEGMENTATION

The consumer demand for more and better services leads to a growth in new health care products (see table 20). The most obvious and important change is seen in various forms of elderly care that flourish in the 1990s: skilled nursing for those with serious illness, custodial and day care for the frail, home support services for people who can't otherwise stay at home, and so on. Expenditures associated with the prevention, detection, and treatment of AIDS also expand. But services expand for all consumers of health care. For example, more effort is expended on preventive care and wellness programs that have a large upfront cost but that are expected to help reduce per person costs in the future. More home testing and home care are available and are partially reimbursed by insurance. Finally, many social problems are redefined as medical ones, with the increased spending becoming part of the health care budget.

Treatment of the mentally ill homeless and of those convicted of drug use are prime examples. Table 18 outlines the new services responsible for almost $100 billion in added health care spending. The biggest gains are in home health and elderly support services of all kinds. Almost $60 billion goes into nursing homes and their offshoots; $17 billion is added to the "other professional" category, which includes home health agencies; and the provision of at-home equipment and supplies increases by more than $20 billion.

Some of the new programs and services are created in response to new consumer demands or as a reaction to cost containment initiatives: the need for postdischarge home care after the imposition of DRGs is one example. It is ironic, but true, that many of the new services and options responsible for overall growth in the system--wellness programs, flexible benefits, and outpatient surgery centers--were originally conceived as cost containment tools. Other programs are generated by provider marketing as health care facilities compete for patients by designing special products and packages. Existing programs are reorganized and emerge as cancer treatment centers, mental health facilities, substance abuse clinics, or women's health facilities. Satellite clinics improve health care access while channeling patients into the parent hospital, and marketing and promotion activities expand to make sure that all potential consumers are aware of available services. For example, between 1985 and 2000, spending on health care advertising quadruples in real terms to over $4 billion dollars. These ads attempt to further raise consumer expectations about the quality and outcomes of medical care. Increasingly, health care is becoming a consumer-driven industry.

Table 20
Service Expansion

	1970	1985	2000
Outpatient Care	MD office Clinic	MD office Ambulatory centers Surgicenters Diagnostic centers	**MD office Ambulatory centers Surgicenters Diagnostic centers Elderly day care Screening services Wellness centers Mental health support**
Inpatient Care	Acute care hospital Long-term care (nursing home, psychiatric, re-habilitation, etc.)	Acute care hospital Long-term care (nursing home, psychiatric, re-habilitation, etc.)	**Intensive care hospital Nursing home Elder residence Rehabilitation Psychiatric**
Home Care	Visiting nurse	Visiting nurse	**Post-discharge care Visiting staff (all levels) Home support services**
Self-Care	OTC drugs Thermometers Medical texts	OTC drugs Diagnostic kits Self-care equipment Diagnostic and treatment algorithms	**OTC drugs Diagnostic/treatment kits Videocassettes and computerized versions of wellness and screening programs Self-care equipment**

BACKING AWAY FROM MICROMANAGEMENT

This expansion in products and spending can take place because of the waning of the cost containment fervor of the late 1980s. Businesses give ground somewhat grudgingly under pressure from their employees who want more flexibility, and from government, which pushes on the retiree benefits side. But business also relaxes health benefits oversight as it realizes that micromanagement outside of its core business is not cost-effective. Once business has made the easy savings by letting providers and employees know it won't give them a blank check, it turns over the responsibility for micromanagement to the employees and the insurers. In addition, the labor shortage caused by the baby bust of the late 1960s and early 1970s has made more generous and flexible benefits a useful tool in attracting and retaining workers. Business is in a position to offer such programs because the economy and U.S. competitiveness have improved. Many companies revamp benefits packages into cafeteria plans, giving employees discretion over both the amount and type of health benefit they select, while the corporate cost of the total benefits package remains fixed.

The packages offered to employees by private insurers stress choice, but choice at a price. As we have seen, most of the options are among types of managed care, including both indemnity products with administrative controls and capitated plans. But even the capitated offerings tend to stress a wider range of services for the same premium rather than a bare-bones version of health care. It also is evident that the lines have blurred between indemnity insurance and managed care in terms of cost. Indemnity plans often are set up like auto insurance, where the consumers pay big bucks for collision. More complete coverage is only available to those willing to pay more out of pocket. Two factors mitigate this control: many people are willing to pay more for care they think is better; and most forms of capitated care must compete in this kind of benefits marketplace: many plans stress their quality, accessibility, and coverage of long-term care and other new benefits more than their price.

Benefits programs are much less likely to be simple group plans than in the 1980s. A cafeteria of benefits is provided for employee choices: coverage for one or for a family, major medical only or a low deductible, rebates for "wellness" behaviors, or higher premiums for smokers. A direct computer link to the insurance company from the employee cafeteria lets workers shift from option to option, learn more about local providers, and survey past bills for errors. Employee benefits in the 1990s are like money market funds in the 1980s--a consumer-oriented financial planning vehicle. Corporations can control the total cost of their benefits plan, while the employee and insurance company manage the individual pieces.

The federal government also gives way to the demand for more health care. Social dissatisfaction with DRGs grows loud enough that nonhospital-based physicians are never included, while hospitals begin to protest being the only providers covered by cost controls. Coverage for long-term care is demanded by many. But the Medicare trust fund is close to insolvency due to the increased demands for care, and the administration knows that a return to unfettered fee-for-service Medicare would break the newly (nearly) balanced budget--at once or in a few years--as the baby boom ages. The chosen solution is to make a modest increase in the deductibles for Medicare on a means-tested basis and to provide catastrophic insurance as a backup. The political trade-off for increasing deductibles is improved coverage for long-term custodial care and home care. This approach seems to resolve the discrepancies between the rich elderly and poor elderly that became so contentious in the 1980s. However, the political clout of the elderly is sufficient to ensure continued election-year adjustments in benefits, and the catastrophic provisions open the door to Medicare coverage of heroic medicine. The "Medicare solution" actually adds fuel to the rapid expansion in total health care spending. State governments choose a variety of reimbursement plans, both for Medicaid and in regulating insurance within their boundaries. Some states choose to follow the federal model; others maintain the rate setting structures that they set up when DRGs were first established. In response to the severe access problems of the mid-1980s, many states mandate certain benefits and require risk pooling to cover the uninsured. These programs remain in place throughout the 1990s.

Both Medicare and Medicaid provide the option of enrollment in capitated plans. Many Medicare recipients opt for enrollment in the late 1980s, but by the 1990s the capitated option is not perceived as necessarily providing better value. Just as the employee has a wide range of competing options, so the poor and the elderly are given some choice. Certain providers concentrate on the "low-ball" market, but they are continually being challenged by state quality assurance boards and are frequently the target of media exposes. Both state and federal governments also withdraw from managing health care supply. Tuition subsidy and medical school budget increases are no longer automatically adjusted for inflation, and competition and deregulation of professionals are encouraged.

The multiplicity of reimbursement mechanisms results in a pluralistic health care system. This patchwork has been facilitated by the spread of sophisticated information systems; rather than uniting and centralizing all payment functions, computers have allowed differing systems to coexist without confusion. Even the idea of group coverage is weakened by flexible benefit plans, where everyone's program is slightly different.

The physical organization of care becomes more decentralized as the 1990s wear on. In the competition for patients, clinics move closer to the patient (company clinics, shopping malls, even into the aisles of discount stores), doctors practice in multiple locations, and house calls by all types of health care professionals become standard. While increasing access to care and minimizing the very real cost to patients of transport and waiting, the multiplicity of venues for care increases the duplication of resources spent on the physical plant. This duplication is part of the vast increase in spending that occurs.

Into the 21st Century

By 2000, health care is a very big business--by far the biggest sector of the economy and the largest identifiable employer. The system is sophisticated, but it is expensive.

The growth in competition for patients has stimulated the development of new services and health care products, increasing the usefulness and benefits of the system to patients. But there are fewer controls on the misuse of noneffective technologies, wasteful procedures, and the duplication of resources in competing providers.

Finally, the doubling of real health care spending has taken place before the largest segment of the population, the baby boom, is in a position to really need it. While early prevention programs adopted in the 1990s may yet mitigate demand on the system in the 2010s, health care spending as a share of GNP will rise ever further unless there is a real restructuring of incentives and systems. By 2000, some health care planners are raising warning signals about the possible shortages of physicians, acute care beds, and the long-term care facilities needed when the baby boom "hits the wall." In the year 2000, no one has a clear idea about how coverage can be expanded and costs contained except for Senator Kathleen Kennedy Townsend who has raised a proposal she calls, "All American Health Insurance." A summary of the environmental and overall health care system changes occurring in Scenario II (and contrasted with Scenario I) appears in Appendix F.

Impact on Physicians

Physicians Face "Tough Choices"

Under the structural changes of Scenario I, physicians experience some dramatic shifts in their roles. While many continue to practice as they always have, an increasing number experience relative economic constraints and less control over practice location and practice style.

After two decades of very rapid expansion, the rate of growth in the number of active physicians finally declines in the 1980s and 1990s, reflecting the leveling of the size of medical school classes in the early 1980s. The rate of increase in the number of active physicians declines from an average of 3.3 percent per year between 1970 and 1985, to 1.5 percent per year between 1985 and 2000. Still, the number of physicians continues to grow each year, and by the year 2000 there are 126,000 more active physicians than there were in 1985 (see table 21). This continues to exert pressure on physicians in their competition for patients.

Table 21
Number of Active Physicians (Thousands)

Year	Number
1970	312
1980	436
1985	511
2000	**637**

Of even greater significance is the changing types of physician practice. Between 1985 and 2000, the number of physicians in independent practice actually falls by about 8 percent although such physicians continue to account for two-thirds of all patient care activity in the year 2000. The number who are salaried or who work in professionally managed groups where they have little control over the financial decisions and limited control on practice standards rises dramatically--from 30,000 to 167,000. This change in practice setting is fostered by three trends: (1) the yearly entry of a large number of new physicians into practice, (2) the increase in the number of female physicians, and (3) the changing practice patterns of older physicians.

On average, each year between 1985 and 2000, about 18,000 new physicians enter practice. Younger physicians find that hospitals or professionally managed groups offer a number of benefits for a physician just starting out: a ready-built patient group, no capital or office expenditures, no marketing or insurance costs, and clearly demarcated hours and responsibilities. Many are willing to accept lower salaries for the lower risk practice setting.

Approximately one-third of current medical school classes are female, and the total share of female physicians rises from 14.5 percent in 1985 to 25 percent in 2000. With more homemaker and child care responsibilities, female physicians are attracted to professionally managed group practices --combining less administrative and marketing responsibilities with greater sharing of off-hour care.

Finally, many older physicians, frustrated by the increased competition, a greater diversity of players, and dwindling rewards, are likely to drift from active practice to research and administrative jobs. Among all doctors (including residents), the percent who are in salaried positions increases from about 33 percent in 1985 to 50.6 percent in 2000 (see figure 20). Table 22 summarizes these shifts in type of practice.

Figure 20
Physicians on Salary (Percent of Active Physicians Who Are Salaried)

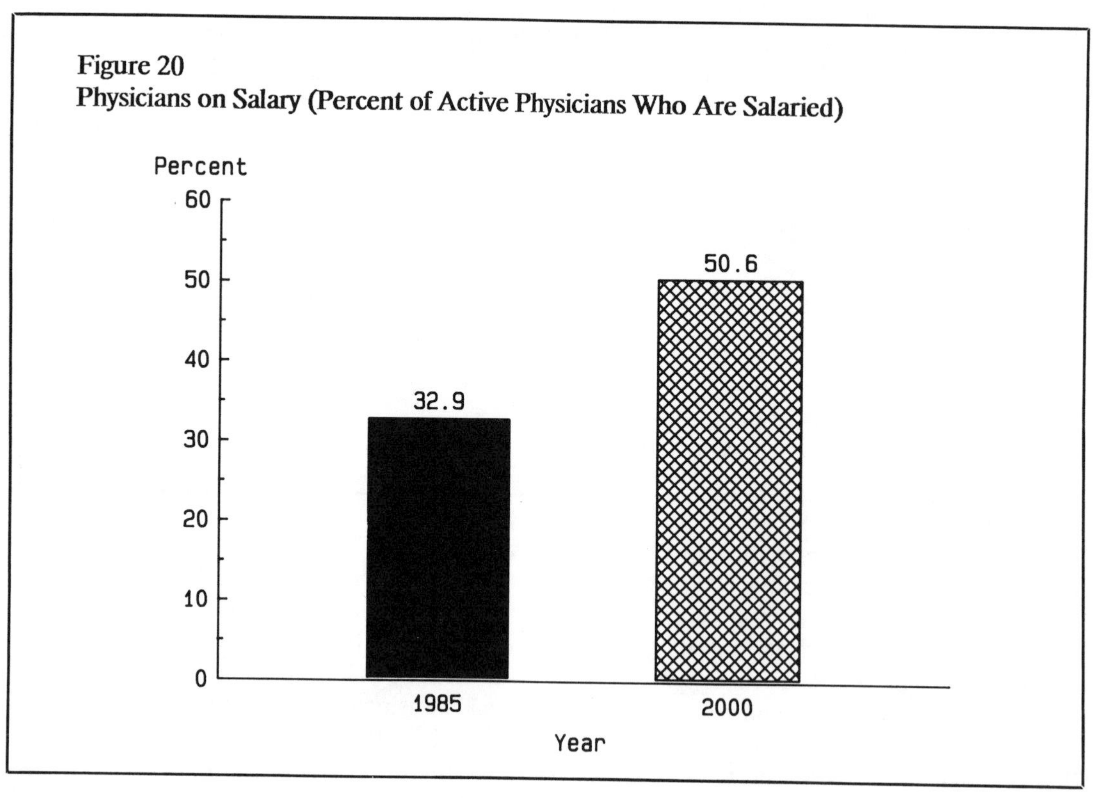

Table 22
Number of Physicians by Major Type of Activity (Thousands)

	1985	2000
Patient care:		
Self-employed	329	306
Salaried/managed	30	167
Total	359	473
Residents	72	66
Administration, teaching, and research	44	61
Federal MDs	22	19
Not classified	14	18
Total active physicians	511	637

Still, the daily activity pattern of many individual physicians remains mixed. A substantial number of physicians in independent offices derive some of their income from contract or capitated care systems through a part-time salaried position at a local hospital or specialized care facility. At the same time, many who work on hospital staffs or in professionally managed groups may receive a portion of their incomes on a fee-for-service basis through some HMO or PPO participation.

The drive to make the health care system more efficient also produces changes in patterns of specialization, although these shifts are gradual in nature. In the period from 1970 to 1985, there was a notable shift from family and general practice to medical and surgical specialties. In the period from 1985 to 2000, general and family practice revives, and other care (for example, diagnostic and psychiatric) grows at the expense of medical and surgical specialties as more attention shifts to ambulatory, outpatient care (see table 23).

Table 23
Physician Specialties (Percent of All Physicians)

	1970	1985	2000
General and family practice	18.7	14.5	17.6
Medical specialties	24.8	31.5	27.4
Surgical specialties	27.7	25.5	24.6
Other	28.8	28.5	30.4

The competitive forces--more physicians, reluctant payers, and the emergence of the management professional--have a dramatic impact on physician income. As more younger physicians go into salaried or managed practice positions, the average income of physicians (excluding federal physicians and residents) actually declines over the period from $113,000 in 1985 to $96,000 in 2000 (in constant 1985 dollars). Still, the total amount of money flowing to physicians continues to increase because of the growing number of physicians and the rising expenses of those running their own office practices (see table 24).

Table 24
Physician Income (Billions of 1985 Dollars)

	1985	2000
Physicians, in Independent Practice:		
Physician income	38.5	30.8
Physician expenses	34.8	35.2
Lab costs/other costs	9.5	15.5
Total revenue	82.8	81.5
Physicians, on Salaries:		
Nonresident MDs	6.9	20.4
Residents	1.8	2.0
Federal MDs	1.6	1.5
	10.3	23.9
Total Revenue	93.1	105.4
Expenses	-44.3	-50.7
Net Income	48.8	54.7

In summary, by the year 2000, medical practice in the United States has undergone some fundamental transformations. The rate of newly licensed physicians and the proportion that are foreign medical graduates have decreased, physicians are less well off economically, about half of all physicians are salaried, and all physicians have experienced a loss of both clinical and economic autonomy. At the same time, physicians also are seeing fewer patients. The result is that the share of health care spending going to the physician sector declines from 22 percent in 1985 to about 17 percent in 2000.

Physicians Under "Health and Wealth"

Under Scenario II, physicians face a more competitive environment than in the 1970s. But to those that adapt, varied opportunities for practice styles abound. In fact, as the pressure for cost containment wanes, physicians breathe a sigh of relief. Many of the terrifying projections of the mid-1980s--such as a drop in real MD income, conversion of doctors to employee status, and a marked loss of clinical autonomy--have not come to pass. Changes in the structure of medical care have expanded services, given physicians more locations in which to practice, raised their real incomes, and left them with control over most of their practices. On the other hand, physicians do not face the golden 1960s again; the 1990s look good only when compared to what might have happened if cost containment had managed to take hold.

Many more doctors are in practice, constraining real physician income growth to 4 percent even as health care expenditures are doubling. Physician expenses increase due to higher practice start-up costs and greater capitalization of the office setting. Also, doctors are forced to manage relationships with insurers and other intermediaries and to market themselves in competition for patients. In addition, physicians have to contend with an increased amount of scrutiny from insurers and more educated consumers, which reduces somewhat their autonomy over clinical and economic practice decisions. For example, physicians receive a flood of utilization and quality review material, ranging from "junk mail" to critical practice inputs from insurers and other intermediaries. Some of the mail comes as "electronic practice profiles," where physicians who are on-line to the insurers for billing and claims processing purposes receive monthly feedback comparing and critiquing their utilization patterns relative to their local and national peers.

By the year 2000, there are 27 percent more active physicians than there were in 1985 (see table 25). Much of this growth occurs in the late 1980s as the last group of baby boom medical students leaves residency programs, but demand to enter a medical career remains high. Physicians retain their prestige and high incomes relative to other professions, and young physicians are perceived to have an enormous growth market open to them as the baby boom ages. Physician retirements from active practice average about 11,000 per year over the period. Although the threats to autonomy and self-directed practice have eased, older physicians find the pace of U.S. health care a little hectic, and they tend to leave active practice when a comfortable lifestyle can be maintained from savings and investments.

Table 25
Number of Active Physicians (Thousands)

Year	Number
1970	312
1980	436
1985	511
2000	**650**

Physician services remain at about 20 percent of health care expenditures, but the growth in total spending means that actual dollars nearly double from about $93 billion in 1985 to over $160 billion in 2000 (in 1985 dollars).

As shown in table 26, there are three components to physician services: (1) net income, (2) expenses, and (3) diagnostic tests performed outside the hospital. Office expenses grow much more rapidly than physician income.

Table 26
Physician Income (Billions of 1985 Dollars)

	1985	2000	Percent Increase
Physician income	48.8	**74.8**	53
Physician expenses	34.8	**70.9**	104
Lab costs/other costs	9.5	**16.7**	76
Total revenue	93.1	**162.4**	74

Net before-tax income rises by 4 percent over the period, after adjusting for inflation, rising from $113,000 in 1985 to $118,000 in 2000. Physicians find that aggressive marketing can help them build and maintain a reasonable practice income, and the demand for specialists in intensive and expensive procedures continues. In fact, income for nonsalaried physicians reaches $135,000; the mean is lower due to the almost 38 percent of doctors who are salaried (including residents). The relative distribution of physicians between general and subspecialty practice remains unchanged from the mid-1980s, largely because of the continued desire of young physicians to pursue specialist careers when they can afford the costs of residency training.

A key change for physicians is the doubling of expenses between 1985 and 2000. While the rapid growth in malpractice premiums slows, the level of malpractice expense is still high. In addition, doctors' expenses for managing their practices and for advertising and marketing themselves among so many other providers increase dramatically. The large crop of new physicians must enter practice and compete in the more heavily capitalized ambulatory environment. The number of practice locations for each physician also increases, so that more equipment and support personnel are needed. Finally, many new office-based diagnostic and therapeutic technologies, which doctors adopt to raise their practice incomes, also have high capital, training, and operating expenses. This is why physician expenses grow so much faster than commercial laboratory spending--many of the new tests bypass centralized labs altogether.

After rising rapidly during the middle and late 1980s, the proportion of new doctors entering salaried positions levels off (see figure 21 and table 27). By 2000, almost 38 percent of physicians are salaried (including residents, administrators, researchers, and those in the federal system), up from 33 percent in 1985. In part this slower growth is due to the reduced enthusiasm for prepaid care (in particular, staff model HMOs), and the slight decline in years of residency training (which reduces the number of residents in the salaried category). Another factor is that many doctors leave salaried practice when they amass enough capital to start or to buy their own practices in the rapidly growing health care system. But many new physicians--particularly the more than 40 percent of new graduates who are women--still prefer a salaried position, one in which an employer assumes the overhead costs. Even self-employed doctors face some reductions in autonomy over the 1980s. The emphasis on both consumer sovereignty and insurer oversight lead to a slight reduction in clinical autonomy and a somewhat larger reduction in economic control (equipment purchase, price setting, and so forth). While a painful change to older physicians, this is an improvement over the threatened environment of rigid cost containment.

Figure 21
Physicians on Salary (Percent of Active Physicians Who Are Salaried)

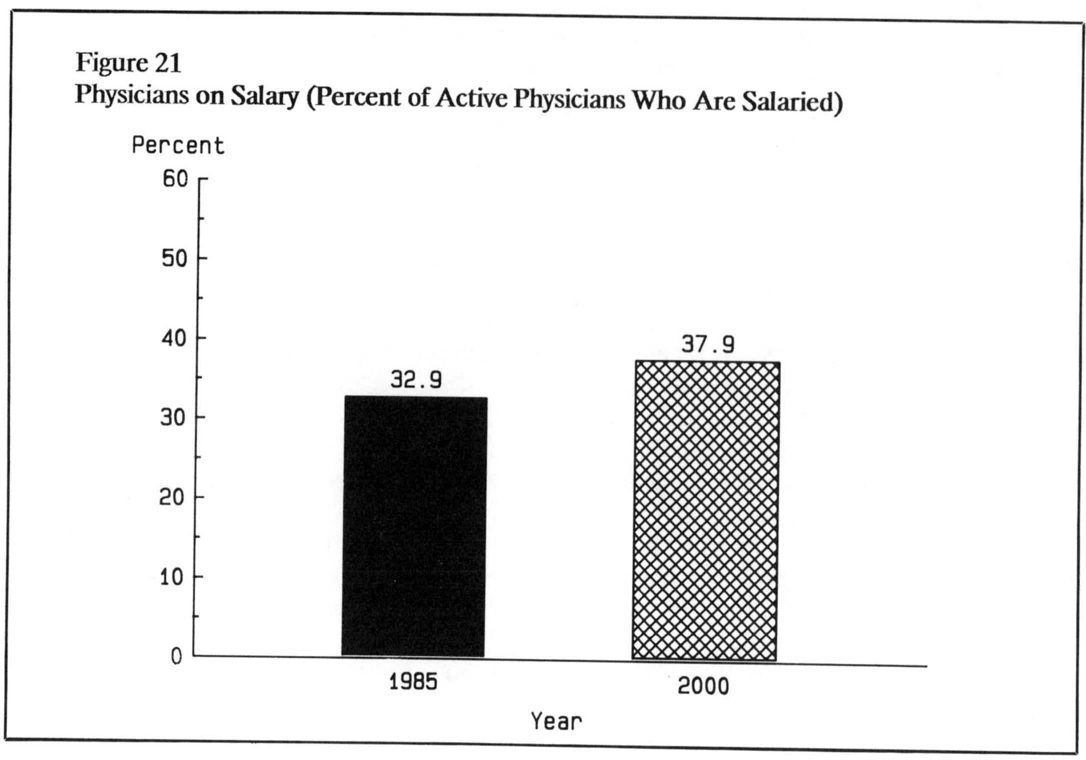

Table 27
Number of Physicians by Major Type of Activity (Thousands)

	1985	2000
Patient care:		
Self-employed	329	393
Salaried/managed	30	82
Total	359	475
Residents	72	72
Administration and research	44	60
Federal MDs	22	25
Not classified	14	18
Total active physicians	511	650

What Does It Mean?

Some common themes for physicians run through both scenarios. The number of physicians rises dramatically as current medical school graduates move into active practice. The greater proportion of females among young physicians and medical school students increases their relative share of practicing physicians over the period. The number of young physicians in salaried jobs increases, and the expenses associated with running a physician's office rise dramatically over the period, putting a greater priority on financial controls. Finally, the ability to adapt to a rapidly changing environment also forces independent physicians to develop expertise in everything from information and technology management to marketing.

The differences between the two scenarios highlight the most important uncertainties that physicians will confront. There is great uncertainty over who pays for the increased expenses of the physician's office--the physician as an independent entrepreneur or some outside organization that can provide capital and management skills. The uncertainty spills over into who will manage the provision of physicians' services, including the types of diagnostic tests given and referrals made. Finally, the choice over control of practice settings is likely to determine the relative income level of younger physicians.

Table 28 (at the end of this chapter) and Appendix F show a summary of comparative physician characteristics for both scenarios. The common themes and the key uncertainties form the basis of the main issues that physicians will face over the period to the year 2000. (See Appendix B--Phase 3: Health Care Scenarios and Issues, for a description of the process used to generate issues.) Nine issues physicians identify as crucial include:

1. Physician surplus. The growth in the number of physicians creates a complex set of problems and opportunities. There will be problems in the growing competition for customers. The problem will be acute for younger physicians just entering practice who may take years to establish themselves in independent practice while carrying large debts from their education. The pressure to secure an income is likely to drive many into salaried positions or group practice. Many young physicians may find that business considerations play an increasing role in deciding not only where they practice but the conditions of that practice as well.

2. Physician autonomy. The drive to secure a regular customer base is driving an increasing portion of young physicians into settings where professional managers will determine the economic conditions of work and even the standards of practice and referrals. While only a minority of practitioners will be in professionally managed settings through the year 2000, an increasing number of patients

will be nonetheless dealing with physicians who have some important constraints on their range of clinical decision making.

3. Practice styles. The push for cost constraint in the health care system creates economic incentives that will lead to major shifts in physician practice styles such as: use of more technologies in the office setting, associations with managed care settings, more response to payer standards, and new niche markets.

4. Physician/hospital relationships. The cost of operating an independent office will force more physicians into managed care settings. The move of more patient encounters to the outpatient setting will shift hospital attention to patients in such settings. In this context, physicians may find that more hospitals use only "closed" or "affiliated" staffs. With the relative advantages that hospitals have in purchasing equipment, setting up liability umbrellas, and marketing, physicians could find the power swinging in favor of hospitals.

5. Physician/government relationships. A basic conflict is gradually emerging in the way government affects physicians' practices. Government is responsible for setting the standards of medical care in the country. Through its roles as the largest purchaser of health care, the largest funder of R&D, and educator and regulator of the system, government seeks to assure a high quality care system for all. At the same time, budget problems are forcing government to push for more cost-effective care for its clientele and to pass on more responsibility to other participants in the system. Physicians often find themselves caught between contrary government pressures for cost effectiveness and quality.

6. Rationing of care. Ten years ago, decisions over what care a particular patient would get were made privately between a physician and a family. Today, these decisions are made in public and may involve the courts, government, and the media. Rationing decisions still must be made, but the loss of a portion of a physician's traditional clinical autonomy makes the decision more complex and time consuming. Ultimately, we may be led to economic tiering where only the rich can afford to buy special care.

7. End-of-life care. A special issue for the physician is the decision over the use of heroic measures near the end of life. With no explicit standards on the application of technology to patients, and with the rising cost of long-term care borne heavily by the family unit, the physician is often forced into ethical and moral choices for which he or she may be ill prepared.

8. Malpractice. An increasing portion of society doesn't want to accept the risks of living in a complex world. In many cases, people use the tort system to seek redress for medical procedures that go wrong. The extent of the phenomenon has two major impacts. First, the size of the premiums for malpractice insurance has become a major burden for doctors in independent practice, and second, the practice of defensive medicine is widespread in many physician practice settings. Both of these factors increase costs and make cost containment efforts difficult.

9. Role of medical associations. As physician performance comes under increasing review not only by peers but by payers, patients, and other agents, the traditional medical associations at county, state, and national levels will be facing new challenges. Should medical associations become more active as quality assurance and credentialing agencies? How should organized medical associations relate to groups of physicians involved in PPO or IPA arrangements? How should these associations relate to state level quality assurance systems? What role should these associations play in dealing with the community at large?

Table 28
Physicians: Comparative Summary of Scenarios

Indicator	1985	2000 I	2000 II
Number of Active Physicians (including federal)	511,090	637,000	650,000
Number of New Physicians Per Year	21,000	17,600	21,000
Average Physician Income in 1985 Dollars (excluding residents)	113,000	96,000	118,000
Percent Physicians on Salary (including residents)	32.9	50.6	37.9
Share of Health Care Spending:			
Billions of 1985 dollars	93.1	105.4	162.4
Percent	21.9	16.9	20.6
Distribution of Income and Expenses (billions of 1985 dollars):			
Physician income	48.8	54.7	74.8
Physician expenses	34.8	35.2	70.9
Lab costs/other costs	9.5	15.5	16.7

Impact on Hospitals

Hospitals Face "Tough Choices"

In Scenario I, traditional indicators of the health of the hospital industry change dramatically as hospitals transform the range of activities in which they participate, the organizational style they adopt, and the contractual arrangements under which they operate. Traditional inpatient indicators drop through 1990: total patient days decline by 30 percent between 1980 and 1990 and then rebound somewhat as the population ages (see table 29 and figure 22). If patient days are measured against a steadily increasing population and an increasingly aged population, we find a decline in utilization of almost 40 percent during the 1980s.

Table 29
Hospital Activity Descriptors

	1970	1980	1985	1990	2000
Total admissions (millions)	29.3	36.2	33.5	28.4	30.7
Length-of-stay (days)	8.2	7.6	7.1	6.8	7.0
Total patient days (millions)	240.3	275.1	237.9	193.1	214.9
	(Per 1,000 Population)				
Admissions	137	160	141	114	115
Patient days	1,121	1,218	1,004	774	805

Figure 22
Hospital Admissions (Millions)

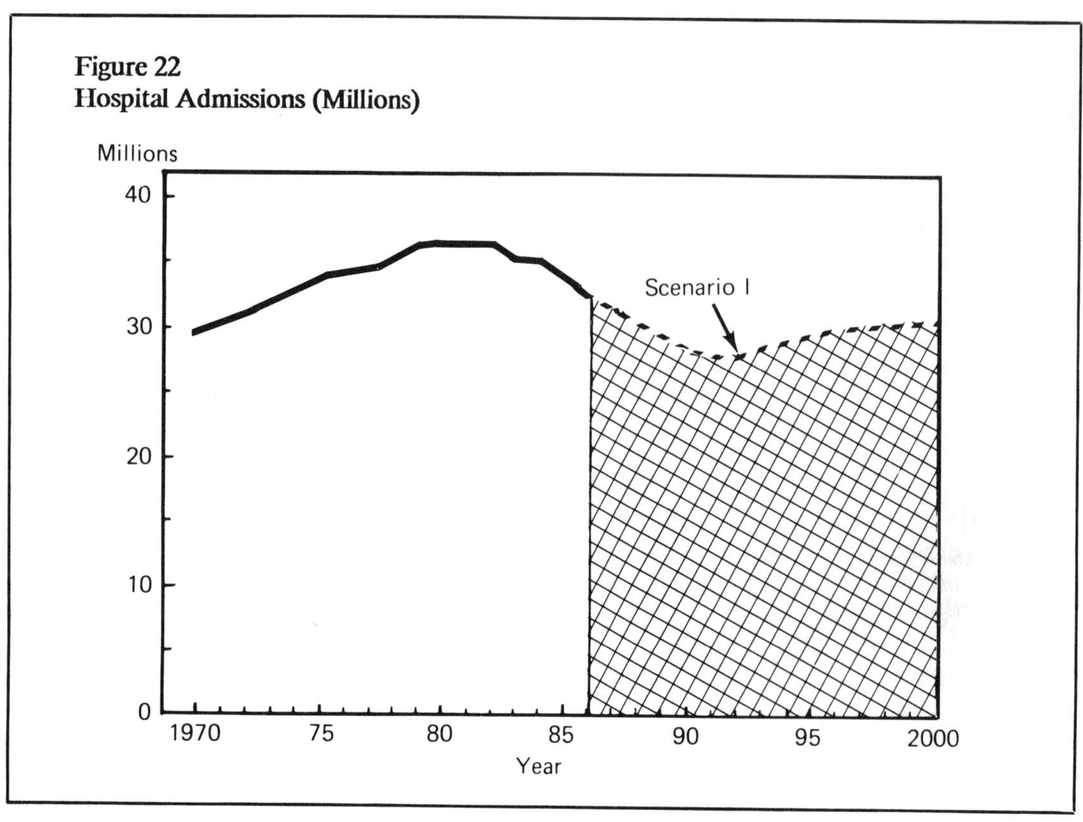

The drop in inpatient activity is a phenomenon that affects all age groups, with a slightly sharper fall for those under age 65. The rate of admissions per person in the over-65 population is about 3.5 times as high as that of the population under 65. Because of the more rapid growth in the number of people over 65, their admissions, which accounted for 29 percent of all admissions in 1985, will account for almost 35% of all admissions in 2000.

While inpatient activities decline in size, outpatient activities grow rapidly. As a percent of all hospital income, outpatient activities grow from 16 percent in 1985 to 31 percent in 2000 (see figure 23). Outpatient activities cover any non-inpatient revenue-producing activities that show up on a hospital's balance sheet. They include such in-hospital outpatient activities as emergency room services, ambulatory care facilities, and outpatient testing. They also include such off-site functions as support and ancillary services provided to other local health care deliverers, sponsored HMOs or associated PPOs, community imaging centers, and testing labs. Even real estate from hospital-owned professional buildings is a new revenue product. While hospital buildings are less central to the health care delivery system than they were in the 1970s, hospital administrators continue to be deeply involved in every aspect of community health care delivery.

Figure 23
Outpatient Revenues (Percent of All Hospital Revenues from Outpatient Activity)

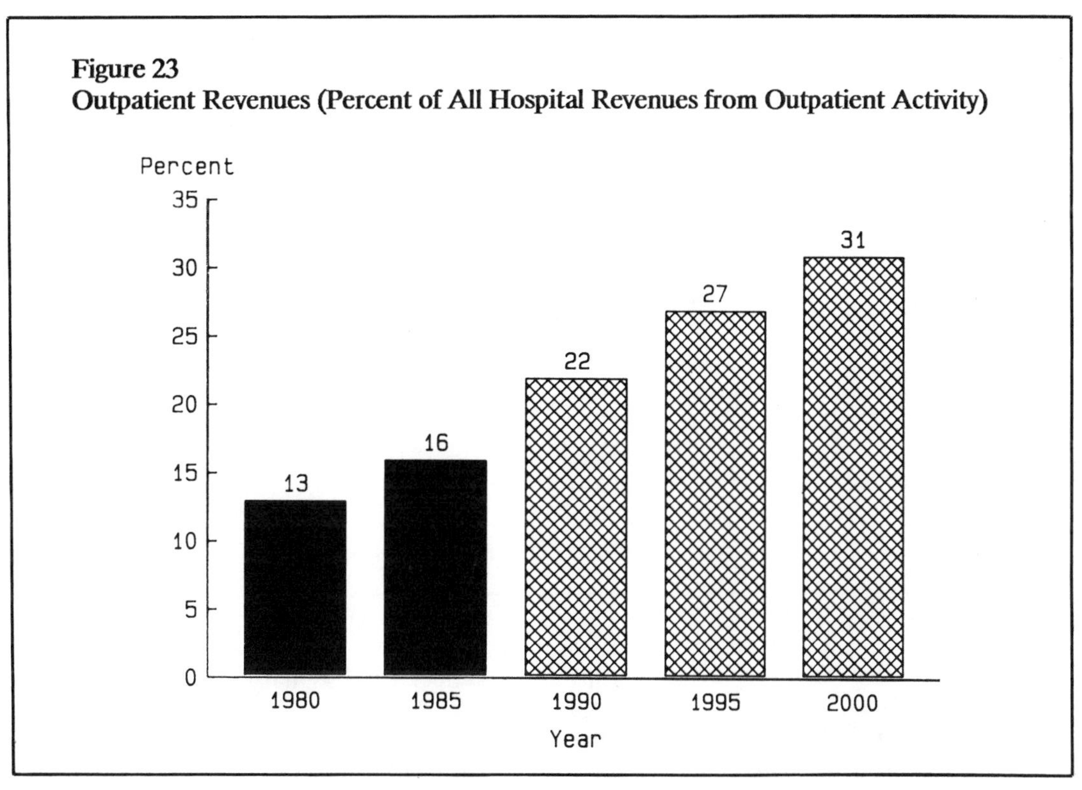

By 2000, hospitals are still centrally involved in health care, but many of them have had to undergo painful transformations in the late 1980s and early 1990s. The drop in admissions and length-of-stay that continued through the latter half of the 1980s forces many hospitals to radically restructure their inpatient services. It becomes apparent in the late 1980s as average occupancy rates approach 60 percent in community hospitals that economic failure is inevitable unless beds are closed (see table 30). As a result, 20 percent of U.S. community hospital beds are taken out of service from the mid-1980s to the mid-1990s. The picture for inpatient care utilization does not start to really improve until the mid- to late 1990s as the aging of the U.S. population begins to have a more marked effect.

Uncompensated care is a problem that is still unresolved despite the rhetoric of health policymakers and the horror stories in the press. By 2000, uncompensated care accounts for 6 percent of hospital revenues, just as it did in the 1980s.

Table 30
Hospital Beds and Occupancy Rates

Year	Number of Community Hospital Beds (Thousands)	Occupancy Rate in Community Hospitals (Percent)
1960	639	74.7
1965	741	76.0
1970	848	78.0
1975	947	74.8
1980	992	75.4
1985	1,003	64.8
1990	**880**	**60.0**
1995	**800**	**70.0**
2000	**818**	**72.0**

The economic pressures on hospitals and the restructuring of inpatient care that results have a profound effect on hospitals with less than 100 beds. By 1985, average occupancy rates for this group fell below 50 percent (with hospitals with less than 24 beds having occupancy rates of 36 percent). This decline continues until hospital administrators realize that managed care is here to stay and that many small, underutilized hospitals in metropolitan areas are simply surplus, and they are closed down entirely. Some other small hospitals in this predicament are brought into the web of influence of larger institutions (both larger hospitals and multiunit alternative delivery systems). These smaller hospitals become satellite clinics, ambulatory care centers, or hospices, but they no longer fulfill a role as hospitals in the conventional sense. These mergers and closures produce a profound change in the distribution of beds in small community hospitals, particularly those in rural areas (see table 31). Since hospitals with less than 100 beds account for 44 percent of all the hospitals in America in 1985, this restructuring affects a very large proportion of hospital administrators and local communities.

Table 31
Beds in Small Hospitals
(Share of All Community Hospital Beds in Hospitals with 99 Beds or Less)

Year	Percent
1985	14.2
1990	12.0
1995	9.0
2000	8.0

The late 1980s and early 1990s are not happy times for the investor-owned hospital chains. They stop expanding in the late 1980s and concentrate on wringing greater efficiencies from their networks. The investor-owned multihospital systems are still in evidence as national entities, but the truly successful players are the multiunit providers who have developed a wide range of services in a particular region. These for-profit actors concentrate on managing resources in particular metropolitan areas, which allows them to generate the kinds of economies of scale achieved in more centralized and regionalized systems such as Canada, France, and the United Kingdom. In most cases, the backbone of these regional systems is a network of local hospitals of varying sizes and specialties.

Community hospitals are only part of the picture. Table 32 shows the change in distribution of total hospital services for 1985 and 2000. The share of total hospital spending going to community hospitals increases slightly from 85 percent to 88 percent as noncommunity hospitals (federal, nonfederal psychiatric) feel the effects of cost containment.

Table 32
Hospitals' Distribution of Total Health Care Spending (1985 Billions of Dollars)

	1985 (Estimated)	2000
Total Hospital Services	156.4	245.1
Community Hospitals:	133.3	215.7
Inpatients	119.5	148.8
Outpatients/satellites	13.8	66.9
Federal	12.3	15.6
Nonfederal Psychiatric	8.3	10.8
Other	2.5	3.0

On balance, the hospital sector appears to have done well over the period. Its share of the health care pie has risen slightly from 37 percent to 39 percent as the hospital continues to play a central role in the management of health care. Expenditures on hospital services have increased by almost $90 billion over the last fifteen years of the century (see table 32). But this apparent rosy picture should be placed in context. From 1970 to 1985, hospital services grew (in real terms) at an average annual rate of 5.1 percent, which was almost exactly twice the real rate of growth in the economy as a whole. However, between 1985 and 2000, total hospital expenditures grow at a rate of 3.0 percent per annum, only a half percentage point better than the economy as a whole. In addition, the restructuring of hospital care leaves the hospital administrator in a difficult position. She has to contend with a more geographically dispersed set of hospital owned and operated facilities, as well as managing a core of very high-intensity inpatient care. (The markedly lower admission rates mean inpatients are very much sicker and more expensive to treat in 2000 than in 1985. Hospital expenditures per acute care admission rise from $3,303 to $4,847 in 1985 dollars.) Hospitals keep moving forward, but the golden age of the 1970s and early 1980s has passed.

Hospitals Under "Health and Wealth"

In Scenario II, hospitals position themselves to serve an aging, affluent, and technologically sophisticated society. Hospitals back out of the attempt to be insurers that was fashionable in the mid-1980s. Instead, large hospitals invest in themselves, striving to become full-service providers; smaller facilities integrate horizontally or try to become niche providers. Most hospitals expand marketing and advertising, create new products and treatment centers, and invest in the latest technology to attract their share of the expanding health care pie.

The sharp reduction in hospital admissions caused by cost containment pressures in the mid-1980s bottoms out in the late 1980s and edges up steadily, reaching 36.5 million in 2000 (see figure 24 and table 33). This trajectory is the result of a number of countervailing forces. First, the rapid growth of managed care in the mid-1980s is the key factor driving admissions down. The rates of hospital use fall precipitiously from 1984 to 1988 as virtually all payers institute some form of control on hospital admissions. By 1988, the easy savings have been made and, although the managed care revolution succeeds in lowering admission rates for those over 65 as well as for those under 65, these prove to be a one-time saving.

Figure 24
Hospital Admissions

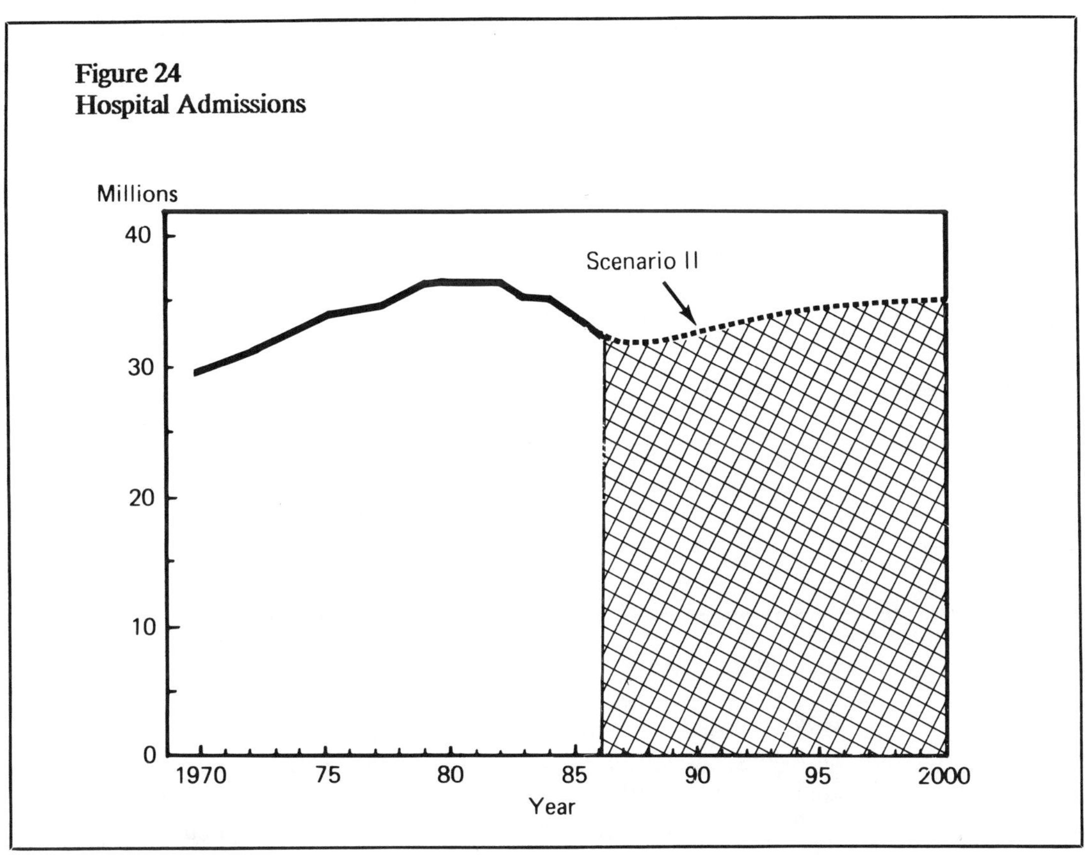

Table 33
Hospital Activity Descriptors

	1985	1990	1995	2000
Total admissions (millions)	33.5	33.7	35.3	36.5
Length-of-stay (days)	7.1	6.8	6.9	7.1
Total patient days (millions)	237.9	229.2	243.6	259.2
	(Per 1,000 Population)			
Admissions	141	135	136	136
Patient days	1,004	923	940	966

By the late 1980s, with the payoff from managed care exhausted, the second key force comes into play: the aging of the population (see table 34). The over 65 population has rates of hospital use 3.0 to 3.5 times as high as the population as a whole. But of particular importance is the rapid growth in the 75- to 85-year-old cohort that has admission rates five to six times as high as the population as a whole, and growth in the over-85 population that has rates of use six to seven times as high.

Table 34
The Aging of the Elderly

Age Cohort	Number (Millions) 1985	2000	Net Increase in Number 1985-2000
65 - 74	17.0	17.7	0.7
74 - 84	8.8	12.3	3.5
85+	2.7	4.9	2.2
Total 65+	28.5	34.9	6.4

The third factor that helps bolster admissions is the broadening of the health insurance net. The uninsured became a major political issue in the 1988 election, and reform in health insurance for the poor and working poor provides hospitals with considerable relief to their problems of uncompensated care (which drops from 6 percent in 1985 to 3 percent in 2000). It also helps bolster hospital utilization as more of the population becomes full participants in the system.

The fourth factor--increasing sophistication of outpatient technologies --is a countervailing force that helps to moderate the rate of growth in hospital admissions so that in the face of a rapidly aging population the total number of admissions per 1,000 population remains fairly stable.

The cost containment period left its mark on the hospital by moving much care to an outpatient basis (see figure 25). As a result, the hospital of the 1990s has a core of high-intensity, high-technology, high-amenity inpatient care. The intensity, sophistication, and cost of inpatient care increases by over 50 percent per admission by 2000 as measured by expenditures per acute care admission, which rise from $3,343 to $5,049 in constant 1985 dollars. Ironically, this pattern is the outcome of efforts in the 1980s to cut total costs by shifting more care to outpatient settings. Patients less seriously ill are spun off into ambulatory clinics or separate nursing units. One result of this reorientation is that residency training for many young physicians moves into alternative sites, giving new doctors a chance to see all types of patients rather than just those in intensive care.

Figure 25
Outpatient Revenues (Percent of All Hospital Revenues from Outpatient Activity)

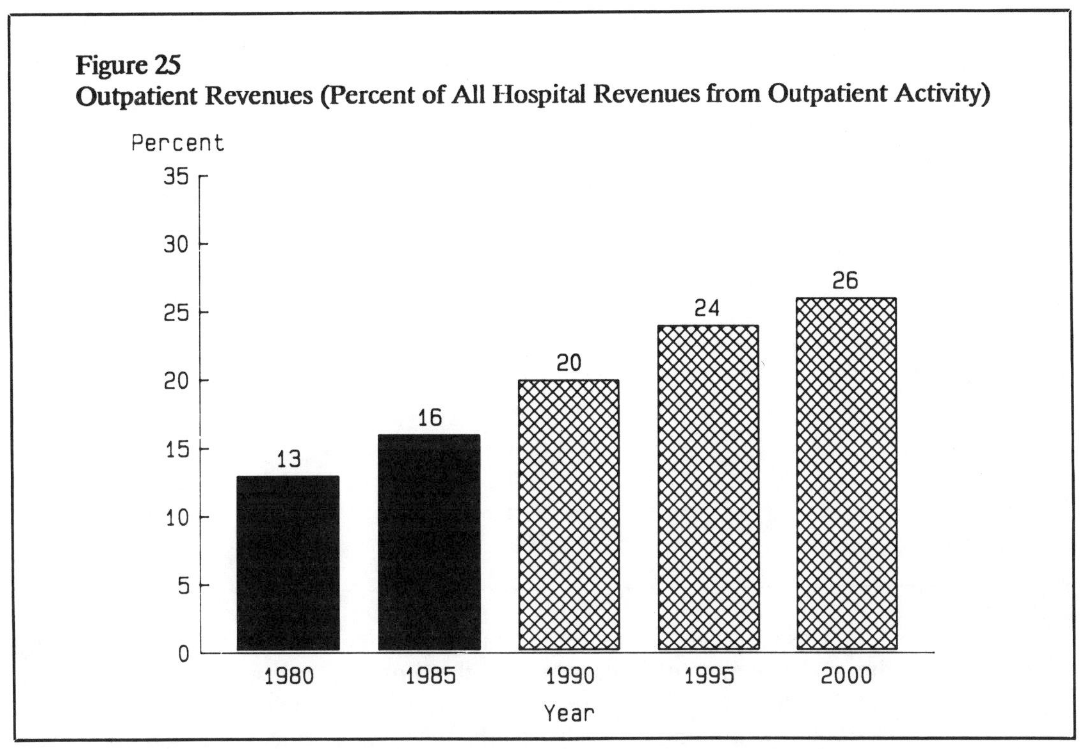

Although the hospital environment is less competitive than feared, it is more competitive than it was in the early 1980s. The squeeze on utilization and occupancy rates continues through 1990, but most hospitals are able to weather the storm (see table 35). However, providers are now profit-maximizing rather than cost-maximizing; that is, making the rate of profit the key figure rather than the amount of revenues. Many hospital products are insensitive to price changes, but insurers still retain some control over what will be reimbursed. And consumers retain some of their skepticism over the costs of terminal care. Small hospitals barely keep their heads afloat, while large hospitals tend to run large profits. On balance, hospital profits average 3 percent to 5 percent of revenues.

Table 35
Hospital Beds and Occupancy Rates

Year	Number of Community Hospital Beds (Thousands)	Occupancy Rate (Percent)
1960	639	74.7
1965	741	76.0
1970	848	78.0
1975	947	74.8
1980	992	75.4
1985	1,003	64.8
1990	**969**	**65.0**
1995	**970**	**69.0**
2000	**1,009**	**70.0**

Hospital care is not a commodity in the 1990s, and, consequently, the major competitive pressure in the hospital industry is in finding the right niche in a highly segmented market. Small hospitals that don't position themselves correctly in this new health care market are swept aside (see table 36). But many small hospitals are successful in repositioning themselves as "boutique" providers, catering exclusively to a particular market segment; for example, arthritics, sports medicine, women's hospitals, drug and alcohol rehabilitation hospitals, or cancer centers.

Table 36
Beds in Small Hospitals
(Share of All Community Hospital Beds in Hospitals with 99 Beds or Less)

Year	Percent
1985	14.2
1990	**12.5**
1995	**11.7**
2000	**11.0**

Many of these "boutiques" are either owned or under exclusive contract to a large, full-service provider who tries to develop a wide ranging portfolio of services that will be attractive to employers, insurers, and, most importantly, individual consumers. Providers who make the transition to a more consumer-oriented health care service find themselves on the edge of a bonanza as the baby boom ages, and several of the investor-owned chains reorganize their focus to compete more effectively as full-service providers in particular metropolitan markets.

The share of the total health care dollar spent in hospitals stays roughly the same through the 1990s at around 37 percent. Although many more kinds of care are offered in other locations, hospital care is the most capital- and skilled labor-intensive, and thus the most costly per patient. These costs increase with the application of new and "half-way" technologies (advances in imaging, biotechnology, transportation, in vitro fertilization, and so on) that society refuses to ration by any means other than the ability or desire to pay. Additional expense is created by the increase in marketing efforts, by raising the amount spent on special programs and promotions, and by offering "hotel functions" such as better food.

Community hospitals are still a very important part of the health care system (see table 37), but they are very different institutions than the hospital of the 1970s. Hospitals, whether profit or nonprofit, are market-oriented and businesslike. The successful hospital administrator in the 1990s has steered his institution through a difficult time but has produced an organization that is responsive to consumer needs for quality and service.

Table 37
Hospitals' Distribution of Total Health Care Spending (Billions of 1985 Dollars)

	1985 (Estimated)	2000	Average Annual Growth Rate
Total Hospital Services	156.4	288.0	4.2
Community Hospitals:	133.3	249.0	4.3
Inpatients	112.0	184.3	3.4
Outpatients/satellites	21.3	64.7	7.7
Federal	12.3	20.0	3.3
Nonfederal Psychiatric	8.3	16.0	4.5
Other	2.5	3.0	1.3

What Does It Mean?

Some common themes for hospitals run through both scenarios. These include an increasing emphasis on ambulatory care and on the organizational and informational linkages between inpatient and other sites of care in the local area; increasing intensity of inpatient care as the hospital becomes the locus of care for the very sick; increasing competition between hospitals and other delivery systems; and increasing pressures to consolidate and rationalize the small independent and underutilized hospital.

The differences between the two scenarios are significant and highlight the uncertainty over the pace of change in U.S. health care. There is considerable uncertainty over the pattern of inpatient utilization, although in both scenarios hospital admissions follow a similar trajectory: continued decline and then moderate recovery as the effects of an aging population take over. The key question is whether the decline in the number of admissions will halt in the late 1980s as all the easy savings of managed care are made, or whether the decline will continue steadily into the early and mid-1990s as cost containment continues. If admissions continue to decline steadily into the 1990s, this will push a larger number of small, underutilized hospitals over the edge, if not into closure then into amalgamation or change of primary function. There also is considerable uncertainty over resolution of the problems of the uninsured and of uncompensated care in hospitals, which again are issues that could force certain vulnerable hospitals into an unsustainable financial position. There is a key uncertainty over which institutional actor/s will govern the health care system and, in particular, how hospitals will fair vis-a-vis patients, payers, and physicians. There also is a considerable difference between the scenarios in the diffusion and use of different types of technology. Finally, there is considerable difference in the degree of vertical and horizontal integration in the system, in particular, whether regionalized health care systems will centralize and eliminate the duplication of services.

Table 38 (at the end of this chapter) and Appendix F show a summary of comparative hospital characteristics for both scenarios. The common themes and key uncertainties underlie twelve major issues facing hospitals. (See Appendix B--Phase 3: Health Care Scenarios and Issues, for a description of the process used to generate issues.) The issues identified as crucial are:

1. Hospital competition. Hospitals in urban areas have competed with one another in the past, but the basis for that competition was for prestige, to be first with new technology, and to attract the best physicians. Declining admissions, new competitors in ambulatory care, HMO and PPO contracts, and closer scrutiny of costs and quality are leading hospitals to compete for survival.

2. Dependence on government. Hospitals are heavily reliant on governmental sources of funding because the beneficiaries of government insurance--Medicare and Medicaid in particular--are heavy users of hospital services. The aging of the population inevitably will increase this share. Similarly, any action on the uninsured question will likely raise government's involvement in funding hospitals. At the same time, business may prove to be the most successful payer group in keeping its employees out of the hospital, thereby increasing the proportion of revenues derived from govern-

mental sources. Hospitals therefore will be increasingly dependent on government for their revenues, which increases the need for hospitals to monitor and influence government policy.

3. Appropriate size/appropriate mission. If in the near future hospital inpatient utilization is on the decline, then hospitals will have to confront the question of the number and size of programs they will offer. Establishing the appropriate size and mission for an institution will depend on analyzing local market factors, determining objectively the program strengths of the institution, and defining a strategic plan for the organization.

4. The limits of diversification. It is becoming obvious that not all hospitals can diversify their way out of trouble. If hospitals diversify beyond inpatient care into other health care activities as it seems likely they must do, they will be facing increasingly stiff competition from other hospitals, physicians, and alternative delivery systems. If hospitals diversify beyond health care activities into everything from real estate and retailing to off-track betting, they face competition from local businesses. Nonprofit hospitals in particular will face increasing legal and regulatory pressure from the small business community, which complains of unfair competition from tax-exempt corporations. Many hospitals have reached, or soon will reach, the limits of diversification as a solution to competition.

5. Mergers and closures. Although mergers and closures of hospitals have been far fewer than predicted, it seems inevitable that more hospitals will have to be restructured or taken out of service. The focus of most of this activity will be concentrated in the small general hospitals below 100 beds in inner city urban areas and in those rural areas that are losing population. Particularly difficult questions for hospital boards and administration will involve mergers of religious hospitals of differing faiths; mergers or closures that leave communities with only one hospital; closures of hospitals that leave a community with a hospital monopoly held by a for-profit provider; and closures of hospitals that result in no health care facility in a rural community.

6. Capital. The hospital industry has gone through cycles in the availability of capital dependent on interest rates, government injections of capital, and the tax treatment of a hospital's capital financing. A number of factors could severely affect a hospital's ability to capitalize in what is likely to be a more capital-intensive industry. The possibility of the elimination of tax-exempt status for bonds issued by nonprofit hospitals would have enormous impact on those institutions. Similarly, the reimbursement of

capital under Medicare is likely to be a continuing issue in the late 1980s and early 1990s. Finally, as mentioned in the mergers and closures issue, redeploying capital from nonprofit hospitals that close will be a major problem in the future.

7. Openness and depth of review. Until recently, hospitals have conducted their affairs in a relatively closed environment. Hospitals were not subject to explicit public scrutiny, although most hospitals participated in external accreditation programs and were accountable to their boards for their level of performance. Increasingly, hospitals are being reviewed in greater depth in terms of both cost and quality; they are being reviewed by more actors (payers, government regulatory agencies, and even consumer groups); and the results of these reviews are being more widely disseminated. The recent release of mortality rates for Medicare patients in individual hospitals is an example of greater depth and openness of review. As more information is moved into more hands, employers, managed care organizations, insurers, and patients increasingly will be comparison shopping among hospitals on cost and quality lines. A key implication of increasing review will be a greater number of legal challenges to the use of cost and quality data and disputes over the ownership of such data. This raises the question of whether the confidentiality of doctor/patient relationships will be invoked as a means of preventing compilation of aggregate hospital performance statistics, and whether patients will have the right to review a hospital's performance records.

8. Hospital/physician confrontation. There are a number of areas in which the relationship between hospitals and doctors could explode. For example, if reimbursement mechanisms were established that effectively let hospitals control all payments for each patient--an umbrella DRG for all care including physician services--this would lead to greater strife between the hospital and its medical staff. Similarly, as care is moved increasingly to the ambulatory environment, the "battle" for patients will intensify between hospital-owned outpatient facilities, the physician office, and the alternate delivery center (urgicenter, surgicenter, and so forth). Confrontation also will occur over the selection, acquisition, and use of technology. Historically, hosptals have had little control over the production function of the hospital--a doctor decides when to admit patients and what kind of care they will receive. The key question for hospitals will be who controls the flow of patients and the pattern of care delivered in hospitals: will it be payers, insurers, government, or physicians? The relationship between hospital and medical staff will become increasingly difficult as competitive pressures build and as managed care becomes increasingly prevalent. Resolution of these issues will depend on hospital CEOs demonstrating

strong leadership in aligning the interests of their institution with those of payers, insurers, patients, and physicians. In many instances, the interests of these groups are so varied that conflict inevitably will result. However, strong hospital/physician relations will likely be a critical factor in determining whether hospitals survive the next five years of structural change and intense competition.

9. Uncompensated care. The plight of the uninsured was a pervasive theme in all levels of the study. But uncompensated care in hospitals is of such crucial importance to small rural facilities, inner city institutions, and large county hospitals that it will be the major issue for these institutions over the next five to ten years. As the hospital sector gets squeezed by managed care, DRGs, and the elimination of cross-subsidy in pricing, the pressures will be extremely intense on those institutions with high levels of uncompensated care. Resolution of the uncompensated care issue is dependent on health insurance reform by government. Although government will not necessarily pay the bill for the uninsured, it is likely it will have to take the lead in providing enabling legislation. It is possible that government intervention will be more active at the state rather than federal level, leading to increasing regional differences in the problems of uncompensated care for hospitals. However, if the federal government takes the lead in mandating employee health benefits, this may go a long way in both alleviating the problems of uncompensated care and eroding regional and local differences.

10. Effective use of medical technology. An increasingly large set of medical technologies will be available in the future. Some developments will enable a greater decentralization of care from the hospital to the clinic, the doctor's office, and the home; others will raise the acuity and complexity of inpatient care. It seems inevitable that technology assessment will become a more central issue for hospitals than it has been in the past, including questions about the use of "heroic" medical technologies, regionalization of high-cost technology, and the role of technology in hospital marketing.

11. Acuity, staffing, and burnout. In both scenarios, the level of inpatient acuity increases by almost 50 percent over the fifteen-year period. This will raise enormous tensions in the daily operation of inpatient care. A shortage of critical care nurses is going to be aggravated by greater malpractice risks for those care givers; by more lucrative and less stressful employment opportunities in utilization review, health care marketing, and nonhealth care occupations; and by the inevitable increase in the complexity of care

associated with new medical technology, drug therapy in particular. In addition, the specter of AIDS will loom larger among health care workers, and many will quit their profession or change their location of practice (whether or not such a decision is rational). Hospital administrators, directors of nursing, and other health professionals are going to face enormous challenges in staffing, in-service education, and employee morale building. It seems probable that real wages in the acute inpatient sector will have to rise further to compensate for these pressures--a reality implicit in the high per-patient-day costs of inpatient care in either scenario.

12. Hospital automation. One potential solution may lie in the use of automation in a wider set of hospital activities: the use of databases and expert systems in such areas as clinical pharmacy and medical records; the increasing use of nursing automation such as point-of-care terminals, "intelligent" drug delivery systems, and prepared meals and supplies; and the much closer integration of financial, clinical, personnel, and marketing information systems in the administration of the hospital. The hospital of the 1990s will be more capital intensive.

Table 38
Hospitals: Comparative Summary of Scenarios

Indicator	1985	2000 I	2000 II
Total admissions (millions)	33.5	30.7	36.5
Admissions per 1,000 (number)	141	115	136
Length of stay (number of days)	7.1	7.0	7.1
Patient days (millions)	238	215	259
Patient days per 1,000 (number)	1,004	805	966
Number of beds (thousands)	1,003	818	1,009
Occupancy rate (percent)	65	72	70
Beds in small hospitals (percent of total)	14.2	8.0	11.0
Inpatient/outpatient revenue split (percent)	84/16	69/31	74/26
Uncompensated care (percent of revenues)	6	6	3
Total hospital services (billions of 1985 dollars)	156.4	245.1	288.0
Hospital share of total health care spending (percent)	36.8	39.3	36.5
Inpatient expenditure per acute care admission (1985 dollars)	3,343	4,847	5,049

Impact on Academic Medical Centers

Academic Medical Centers Face "Tough Choices"

In Scenario I, the priority given to medicine in an aging society and the pressure to restrain government spending at all levels are the contrary environmental forces that influence the nation's academic medical centers. The strong political support for medical care makes it extremely difficult for any state to close down an existing medical college. A few consolidations take place, and no new medical schools open, leaving on balance slightly fewer schools in the year 2000 than in 1985 (see table 39).

Table 39
Number of Fully Accredited and Provisionally Accredited U.S. Medical Schools

Year	Number
1970	103
1975	114
1980	126
1985	127
1990	**127**
1995	**124**
2000	**120**

But economic and demographic pressures do have an impact. The number of applicants to medical schools falls sharply from its high point in the late 1970s as the number of individuals in the 20- to 24-year-old cohort drops. Medical schools find that it makes more economic sense to reduce the size of the incoming class than to allow the applications to acceptance ratio to fall much below 1.7 (see table 40). The leveling off in both the application rate and the applicant/acceptance ratio implies that there is no significant decline in the quality of students.

Table 40
Applicants and Acceptances to Medical Schools

	Target Cohort 20-24 Years of Age (Millions)	Number of Medical School Applicants (Thousands)	Applicants per 1,000 Target Population	Accepted Applicants (Thousands)	Applicant/ Acceptance Ratio
1970	17.2	25.0	1.5	11.5	2.2
1975	19.5	42.3	2.2	15.4	2.8
1980	21.6	36.1	1.7	17.1	2.1
1985	21.2	32.9	1.6	17.2	1.9
1990	**18.4**	**29.0**	**1.6**	**16.8**	**1.7**
1995	**17.1**	**27.5**	**1.6**	**16.3**	**1.7**
2000	**16.9**	**27.0**	**1.6**	**15.7**	**1.7**

The drop in the number of acceptances gradually works its way through to the number of medical school graduates and newly licensed physicians (see figure 26). The number of graduates falls by 10 percent between 1985 and 2000. But the declining applicant pool (and the concomitant fall in the acceptance ratio) means that far fewer qualified American graduates of foreign medical schools (FMGs) are applying for licenses each year. Both the number of FMGs and their share of newly licensed physicians decline through the year 2000, from 23.1 percent of new licenses in 1985 (some 4,900 FMGs) to 16.5 percent of new licenses in 2000 (2,900 FMGs).

Figure 26
Newly Licensed Physicians (Total Number of New Physicians Licensed Each Year)

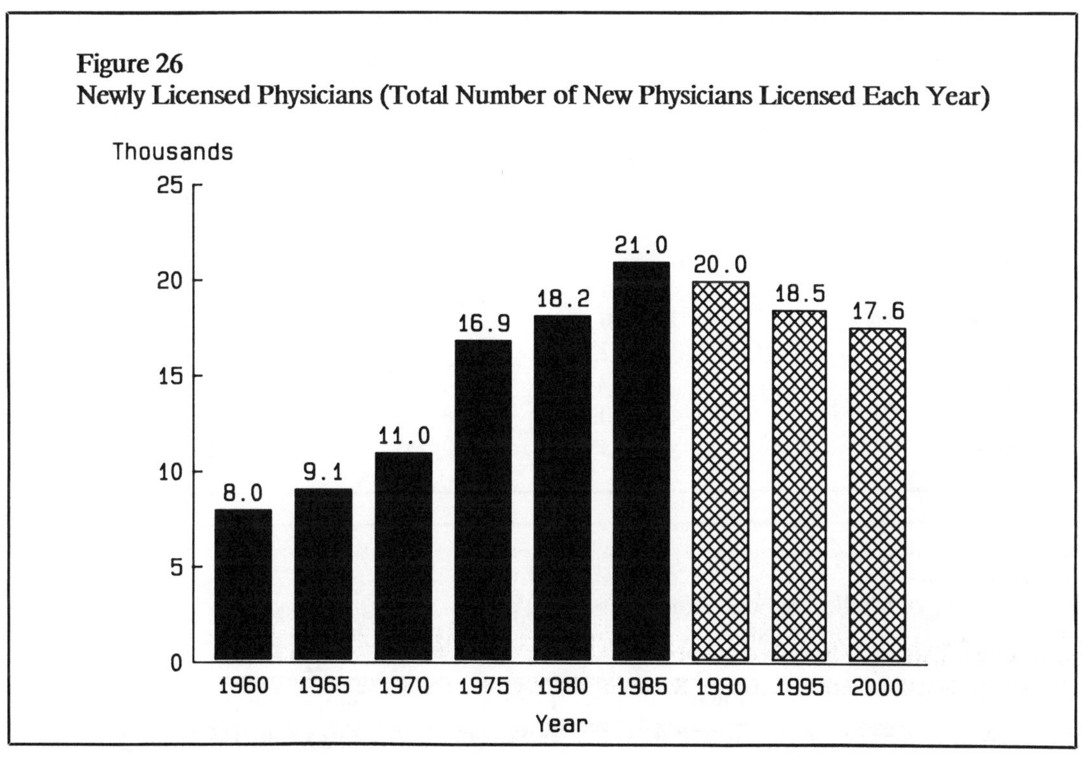

The income of medical schools continues to expand in real terms, averaging 1.4 percent growth per year between 1985 and 2000 (see table 41). This is still less than the overall real growth of 2.6 percent per year of total health care spending. The medical schools lag general growth in the health care sector as government payments for medical education reflect the declining number of students. As table 42 shows, the medical schools continue to increase their reliance on their own resources; that is, income from tuition and fees, research contracts, and hospital income.

Table 41
Medical School Income

Year	Billions of 1985 Dollars	Average Annual Percent Increase over Period
1960	2.5	--
1965	4.4	11.7
1970	6.0	6.4
1975	8.2	6.5
1980	9.7	3.4
1985	11.0 (est.)	2.5
2000	**13.3**	**1.4**

Table 42
Sources of Medical School Funds (Percent)

Year	Own Revenues	Federal Government	State and Local Government	All Other
1960	12	42	19	27
1970	14	45	23	18
1980	33	29	25	12
1985 (est.)	41	24	23	12
1990	**42**	**24**	**23**	**11**
1995	**43**	**23**	**23**	**11**
2000	**44**	**23**	**22**	**11**

The growth in "own revenues" indicates that the patient activity of the teaching hospitals remains fairly competitive. In fact, the specialized acute care resources of the teaching hospitals serve them well through the 1990s. Group practices are not able to compete in complex tertiary care unless their patient population reaches very large numbers (probably on the order of 200,000 people), thus justifying the type of specialization that can be found in the teaching hospitals. In all, the teaching hospitals' share of the number of total inpatients rises. In contrast, the teaching hospitals are less aggressive in investing capital in outpatient or off-site activity, and their share of such activity falls slightly as they find it difficult to compete on price (see table 43).

Table 43
Share of All Patient Activity in Teaching Hospitals (Percent)

Year	Inpatient Days	Outpatient Visits
1975	18.7	28.5
1980	20.1	30.3
1985 (est.)	21.4	30.0
1990	**21.9**	**28.5**
1995	**22.2**	**29.0**
2000	**22.4**	**28.9**

On the research side, the National Institutes of Health (NIH) continues to argue effectively before Congress that biotechnology and medical research are important for the nation's health and international economic leadership. Even though an increasing portion of this research is funded by commercial enterprises and philanthropic organizations, such arguments are able to ensure that public funding grows only slightly slower than real GNP (see table 44). As private sources of research funding become more prominent, more money is channeled to the larger and better funded schools and departments. Whereas the top twenty medical schools accounted for 50 percent of all research funding in 1985, by 2000 they account for 56 percent of the total (see figure 27).

Table 44
Research Spending on Noncommercial Biomedical Research

Year	Percent of GNP	Billions of 1985 Dollars
1980	0.21	7.5
1985	0.19	7.6
1990	**0.19**	**8.6**
1995	**0.19**	**9.7**
2000	**0.18**	**10.4**

Figure 27
Research Concentration (Share of All Research Activity in Top 20 Schools)

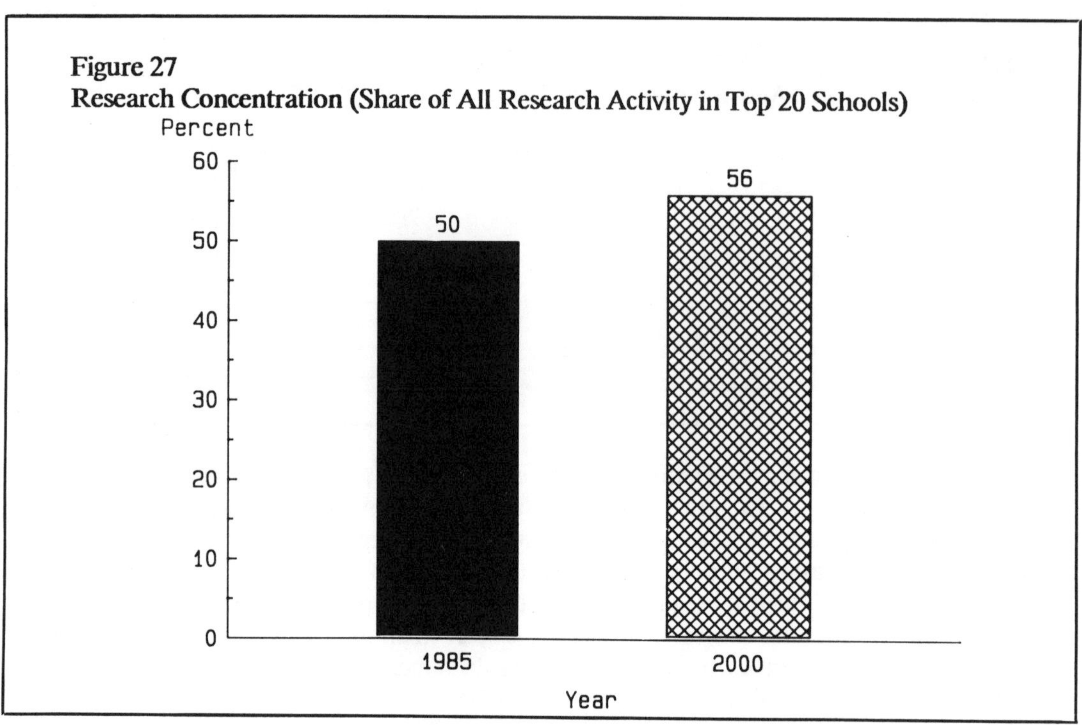

The U.S. medical education system is not suffering unduly, but it is not uniformly excellent; it has a number of institutions that are struggling for survival, and the golden age of the 1960s seems a long way off for faculty in many of the second-tier schools. In these institutions, the dream of a balance among teaching, service, and research has been severely tarnished by fiscal constraints, commercialization, and the realization that they are no longer equal partners in academic medicine.

Academic Medical Centers Under "Health and Wealth"

In Scenario II, the cost containment world of the mid-1980s led to serious reconsideration of the role of the academic medical center. As a result, many attitudes and programs were changed in ways that lasted long after the cost containment effort was dead. Some of graduate medical education follows patient care out of the hospital, and some second-tier medical schools are sold to for-profit providers.

Academic medicine weathers the storms of cost containment and is ready to play a role in the expansion of health care delivery in the 1990s. The group as a whole is held back by the performance of some inner-city medical schools that still have problems of uncompensated care and smaller NIH budgets.

The overall size of the medical education system as measured by number of schools and total enrollment reaches a steady state in the 1980s (see table 45). After a period of rapid expansion in the 1960s and 1970s, the flows through the system level off. There are two principal reasons for the lack of growth. First, there is widespread belief that too many physicians had been produced and that the rate of production should not be increased. Second, the demographic reality of the baby bust generation of the late 1960s and 1970s, who represent a smaller demographic pool of potential applicants, begin moving through the system (see table 46).

Table 45
Medical Students and Medical Graduates (Thousands)

Year	Total Enrollment in U.S. Medical Schools	Total Number of Graduates of U.S. Medical Schools
1960	30.3	7.0
1965	32.8	7.6
1970	40.5	9.0
1975	55.8	13.6
1980	65.2	15.7
1985	66.6	16.1
1990	**66.7**	**16.2**
1995	**67.0**	**16.4**
2000	**67.5**	**16.8**

Table 46
Applicants and Acceptances to Medical School

Year	Target Cohort 20-24 Years of Age (Millions)	Number of Medical School Applicants (Thousands)	Applicants per 1,000 Target Population	Accepted Applicants (Thousands)	Applicant/ Acceptance Ratio
1970	17.2	25.0	1.5	11.5	2.2
1975	19.5	42.3	2.2	15.4	2.8
1980	21.6	36.1	1.7	17.1	2.1
1985	21.2	32.9	1.6	17.2	1.9
1990	**18.4**	**30.3**	**1.7**	**17.0**	**1.8**
1995	**17.1**	**30.0**	**1.8**	**17.1**	**1.8**
2000	**16.9**	**31.3**	**1.9**	**17.2**	**1.8**

These factors mean that the decline in the number of applicants to medical school, which started in the mid-1970s, continues into the mid-1990s. But the relative popularity of medical schools increases again among the cohort of potential students in their early twenties as reflected in the ratio of applicants to population in that cohort (see table 46). Medical students in the 1990s--more than 40 percent of them women--are attracted by the longer term prospects for health care in the next century and by the continued progress and the exciting opportunities for research and patient care offered by new medical technologies. The net results of these changes is a stabilization in the flow of new physician graduates (see table 45).

The average medical resident spends 10 percent less time in postgraduate programs in 2000 than in 1985. This is the case even though there is an explosion of new complex technologies being used and a great deal more money in the system. The reason for the reduction is that the individual student is responsible for a larger proportion of training costs: medical training subsidies from the government are lower, residency salaries don't rise quickly, and research grants are more directly targeted to a few large AMCs with outstanding reputations and a major program focus. As a result, a two-tier pattern emerges among new doctors: "superspecialists," who are more likely to come from white, upper-income groups, and to be male; and physicians with shorter (and cheaper) residency programs who are more likely to be women and minorities.

Overall, with the slowdown in the flow of new medical students, the difficulties of foreign medical graduates securing residency positions in the United States, and the changes in the length and cost of residency training, the number of newly licensed physicians in the United States plateaus through the 1990s (see figure 28). The rate is still high because medicine is still perceived as both a noble and lucrative profession.

Figure 28
Newly Licensed Physicians (Total Number of New Physicians Licensed Each Year)

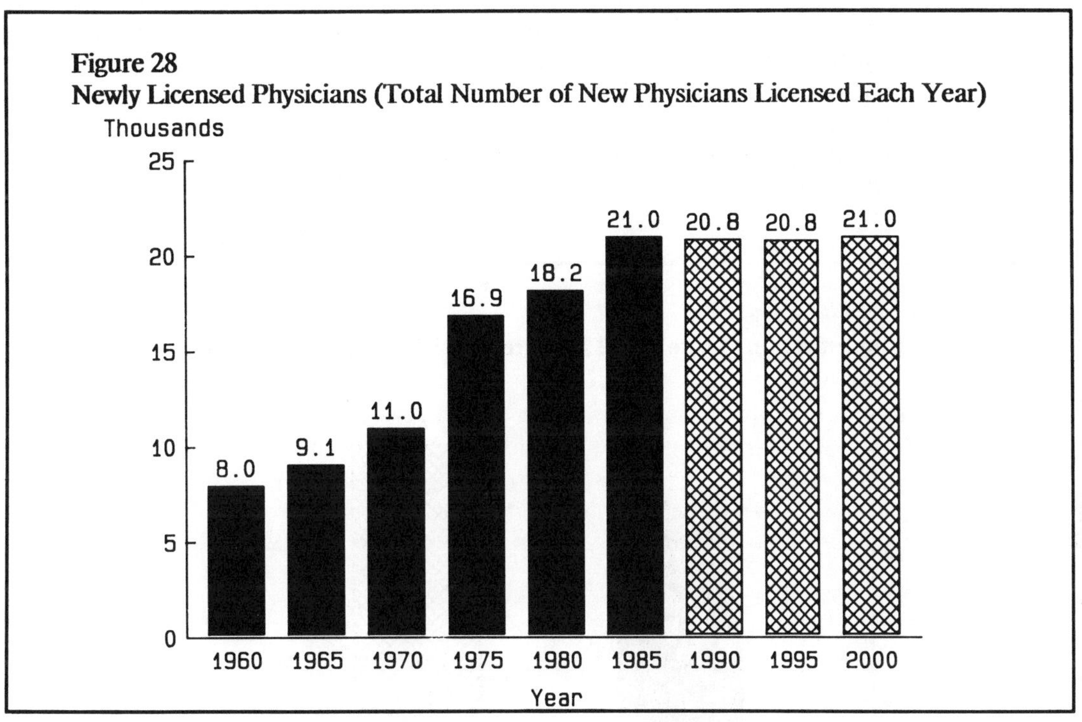

Government spending for medical R&D remains high, but not just as an aid to the health care sector (see table 47).

Table 47
Research Spending on Noncommercial Biomedical Research

Year	Percent of GNP	Billions of 1985 Dollars
1980	0.21	7.5
1985	0.19	7.6
1990	**0.19**	**8.8**
1995	**0.19**	**10.2**
2000	**0.20**	**12.5**

The United States consistently runs a trade surplus in drugs and medical equipment. That surplus shrinks in the mid-1980s, but continued advances in new products restores U.S. competitiveness, and regulatory changes that encourage drug exports restore the trade surplus for this sector. U.S. drug and medical equipment manufacturers continue to invest heavily in R&D as health care supplants defense as the key user and often the key originator of high technology. NIH budgets are increased partly to support technology dissemination through academic medicine and partly to maintain U.S. research leadership in medical technology in general, and biotechnology in particular. However, the distribution of these funds increasingly favors the premier academic institutions as measured by the percentage of all research funding going to the top twenty medical schools, which increases from 50 percent in 1985 to 56 percent in 2000 (see figure 29).

Figure 29
Research Concentration (Share of All Research Activity in Top 20 Schools)

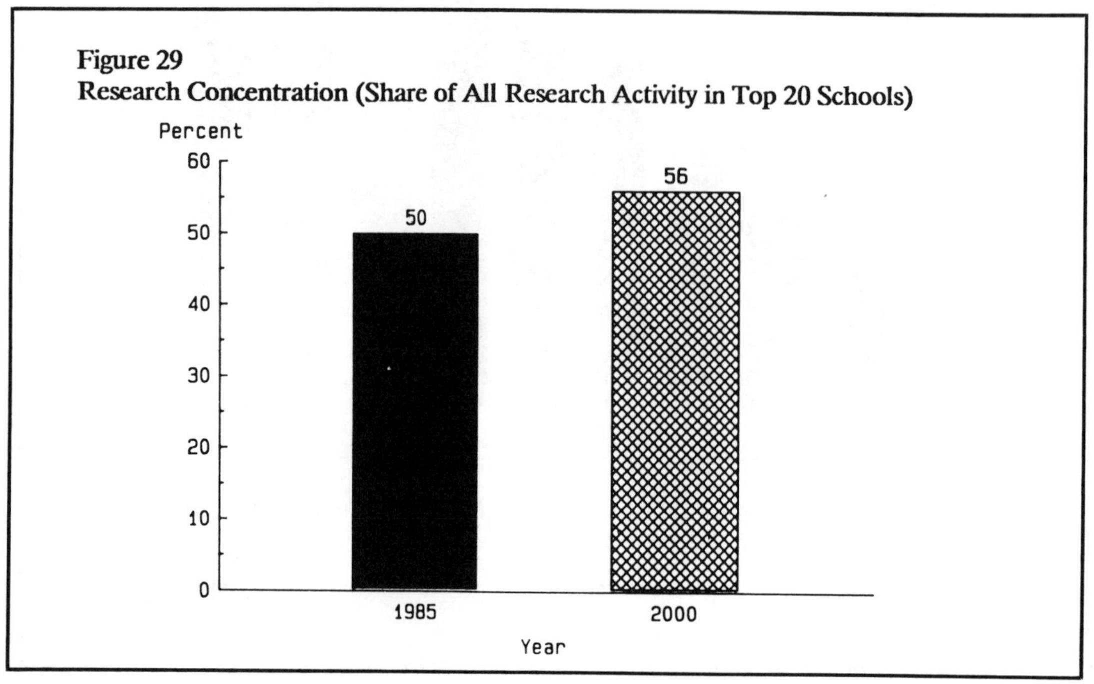

More money is being spent on the medical education system, but the rate of increase has slowed (see table 48). The rapid expansion in funding in the 1970s weakens considerably in the early 1980s and rebounds slightly over the remainder of the century. But the medical education system consumes more real resources each year because of the complexity of the subject matter (requiring greater instructional and research resources per student) and the sophistication of the technology employed in teaching, research, and service activities. Medical schools continue to derive the largest share of income from their own service activities, tuition fees, and so forth (see table 49).

Table 48
Medical School Income

Year	Billions of 1985 Dollars	Average Annual Percent Increase Over Period
1970	6.0	6.4
1975	8.2	6.5
1980	9.7	3.4
1985 (est.)	11.0	2.5
1990	**12.6**	**2.7**
1995	**14.6**	**3.0**
2000	**17.4**	**3.6**

Table 49
Sources of Medical School Funds (Percent)

Year	Own Revenues	Federal Government	State and Local Government	All Other
1960	12	42	19	27
1970	14	45	23	18
1980	33	29	25	12
1985 (est.)	41	24	23	12
1990	**42**	**23**	**23**	**12**
1995	**43**	**23**	**22**	**12**
2000	**44**	**23**	**22**	**11**

The continued financial dependence of academic medicine on its service activities makes the teaching hospital's ability to compete for patients an important element in determining the financial health of medical education. The teaching hospitals are successful in capturing a greater share of inpatient days because of their focus on high technology for the very sick (which is increasingly the rationale for a hospital admission); their location in cities with an older population; and their reputation for quality among referring organizations (see table 50). However, they have difficulty competing on price because of the overhead of teaching functions and uncompensated care. The latter problem is very much ameliorated by the Medicaid reforms and risk pooling legislation of the late 1980s, which helps many inner-city teaching hospitals alleviate their uncompensated care problems. On balance, by the year 2000, patient days increase by approximately 20% from the lows of the late 1980s.

Table 50
Share of All Patient Activity in Teaching Hospitals (Percent)

Year	Inpatient Days	Outpatient Visits
1975	18.7	28.5
1980	20.1	30.3
1985 (est.)	21.4	30.0
1990	21.4	30.3
1995	22.3	29.5
2000	23.3	29.4

In the more dynamic outpatient environment, the teaching hospitals are less competitive. The decline in share of outpatient visits continues, but this decline in share is more than compensated for by the increase in total outpatient activity. Again, the net result is an increase in outpatient visits of over 20 percent between the late 1980s and the end of the century.

The medical education system has survived and prospered in the 1990s, which puts it in a relatively sound position to produce the health professionals needed to take on the biggest challenge of the new century: health care for the baby boom.

What Does It Mean?

The scenarios outline two possible worlds for academic medicine. Some trends are similar in either scenario: the decline in the demographic pool of applicants to medical schools; an increasing proportion of female medical students and graduates; a reduction in the length of postgraduate education; an increasing concentration of research dollars in the elite schools; greater difficulty of teaching hospitals in keeping their share of the outpatient market; and continued reliance on the activities of the university's own resources including medical practice and hospital income as well as tuition for the financial support of medical schools.

Very significant differences between the scenarios do exist, however, which reflect key uncertainties in the environment of academic medicine. These include: uncertainty over the level of support for medical education generally; questions over the relative role of public versus private sector biomedical research and the level of financial commitment by either group to academic medicine; uncertainties over the popularity of medicine as a career and the long-run consequences for quality of care; and, lastly, uncertainties in the overall number of students and graduates that will flow into and out of the system in the next two decades.

Table 51 (at the end of this chapter) and Appendix F show a summary of comparative statistics for academic medical centers for both scenarios. (See Appendix B--Phase 3: Health Care Scenarios and Issues, for a description of the process used to generate issues.) These common themes and key uncertainties serve as a backdrop to ten key issues for academic medicine:

1. Paying for medical education. In any scenario, there will be a continued policy debate over how medical education should be paid for. Individual students will face higher personal financial burdens and more may be drawn into long-term employment contracts as a means of funding medical school and residency training. The medical schools themselves will continue to rely heavily on what they generate through their service activities and tuition fees with only the elite 25 percent of schools having the luxury of healthy government research support. The key role of state governments in funding medical schools will place many second-tier schools at the mercy of their regional economies.

2. Clinical/academic trade-offs. The three foundations of academic medicine--clinical service, teaching, and research--are being pressured in a variety of ways. A clear implication is that increasingly there will be conflict between the service and academic objectives of academic medical centers. Service activities will continue to be a major source of revenue for the medical school, and the competitive pressures faced by hospitals and physicians more generally will be particularly acute for the academic medical center's outpatient activities. Although it is likely that AMCs will fare well in the complex tertiary care market, even there the academic component of inpatient care in a teaching hospital will come under increasing scrutiny. Another area of potential conflict will be between the deans of medical schools and the CEOs of major teaching hospitals. Many of the prestigious university teaching hospitals--although relatively prosperous in economic terms--will be fraught with interorganizational conflict. Other conflicts may emerge over the role of income-generating subsidiaries such as drug and alcohol clinics, utilization reviews of the practice of interns and residents, or the selection of new medical faculty.

3. Town and gown. As the service component of academic medicine receives increasing emphasis due to economic necessity, a greater level of contentiousness will develop in most centers between faculty and nonfaculty physicians. Conflicts will arise over departmental budgets, admitting privileges, and teaching duties. These conflicts will exaggerate the tension between medical school deans

and CEOs of teaching hospitals as a "them-and-us" division emerges between physician groups in many teaching hospitals. The chiefs of medical staffs in teaching hospitals will be put under increasing pressure by these changes, testing their leadership and conciliation skills to the maximum. The division between town and gown may lead to power battles that remove certain teaching hospitals--particularly those with only a few residency positions--from the orbit of the university.

4. Medical school curriculum. As health care continues its transformation, the medical school curriculum increasingly will become an area of contention. Many actors--hospitals, HMOs, and alternative delivery systems--will be pushing for new types of physicians, such as gatekeeper generalists, gerontological general practitioners, and physicians with management, organizational, and even business training. At the same time, within academe, the expansion of knowledge and the associated subspecialization of skills and technology will act to fragment the curriculum and continue the push toward specialization. One particular area of contention will be clinical experience: should physicians receive more of their clinical experience in ambulatory clinics, surgicenters, or even nursing homes, or is a hospital-based tertiary system the best training for physicians to teach them to deal with any eventuality?

5. Medicine and other health professionals. A key set of questions centers around the role of universities in training other health professionals and the potential conflicts between medical schools and schools of nursing, social work, dentistry, pharmacy, public health, health planning, and administration. These debates will be over manpower requirements, resource allocation, and the interaction of health professionals both during and after their training.

6. Women in medicine. The growth in women's participation in medicine has been viewed generally as a positive thing. However, this trend raises several important concerns and implications for the health care system, the number and type of health professionals, and the role and status of women. For example, in 1987, for the first time a survey of female college graduates showed that more were planning a career in medicine than were planning a career in nursing. Women no longer are restricted to a subset of occupations, and many of those interested in health care are choosing to pursue a medical career. This trend creates a number of important effects. One implication is that it may aggravate the nursing shortage as the pool of interested candidates shrinks. A second important implication concerns the dynamics of nurse/physician relationships. In the past, the stereotypical interaction was between the dominant, highly paid male and the subordinate,

poorly paid female. As the sophistication of hospital nursing continues to increase and as the shortage of skilled nurses gets more acute, it seems likely that salaries will be bid up. At the same time, financial pressures on the delivery system and the perceived surplus of physicians are likely to bid down the income of young doctors, a larger proportion of whom will be women. The stereotypical relationship will be transformed as a result, perhaps leading to more consensual decisionmaking among health care professionals. Finally, a key uncertainty for the payers is whether young physicians, in general, and women physicians, in particular, will be more accepting of salaried employment and more constrained working conditions in the future.

7. Funding of biomedical research. A key question is the funding of biomedical research; in particular, the level of funding for basic versus applied research. Government NIH budgets have done well in recent years, but the question remains: will the public continue to support such a national emphasis on research over development?

8. Commercialization of science. A key related issue is the increasing importance of the private sector in science and the blurring of boundaries between university-based biomedical research and the commercialization of biotechnology. The role of pharmaceutical and medical products companies in R&D is likely to increase, and links between academic science and commerce will be strengthened both in the United States and abroad. But such a trend creates difficulties for academic medicine in administering grant programs, attracting certain faculty without giving them an option for privatization of their research, and orchestrating the free flow of new knowledge through academic literature. The ethical and economic questions surrounding research in the academic medical center will be more complex and more contentious.

9. Clinical researchers. A further research administration problem will be in trying to preserve and, if possible, revitalize the role of the MD clinical researcher. The quintessential academic physician was once considered to be the rennaissance character who gave exciting lectures on basic pathology, was an expert clinical instructor, had compassionate and effective clinical skills, and could lead and administer a Nobel prize winning research team. The complexity of medical knowledge and technology and the economic and organizational pressures on teaching and service are making this vision impossible. Yet, there continues to be a need for clinical researchers who blend medical and scientific skills, particularly in the 1990s when a whole raft of new drugs, devices, and scientific tools will reach a critical stage.

10. Fragmentation and tiering in academic medicine. The final issue for academic medicine is really a composite of the other nine. Across a number of dimensions, academic medicine is likely to be more fragmented and more heavily tiered than it has been in the past. In particular, a bigger gap will develop between the top tier medical schools and the rest in terms of budgets and academic missions. Sharper divisions will emerge between those who will have access to medical education generally and those having access to more lengthy high-cost subspecialty residency programs. The disparity in the quality among medical schools in different parts of the country and among those with varying degrees of commitment to academic versus service missions may grow wider. This is likely to lead to a wider differentiation in the quality of physicians produced by the system in the 1990s. Finally, the increased fragmentation and tiering of academic medicine will present substantial challenges for the AAMC itself in representing the interests of such a divergent group.

Table 51
Academic Medical Centers: Comparative Summary of Scenarios

Indicator	1985	2000 I	2000 II
Number of U.S. medical schools	127	**120**	**127**
Number of medical school applicants (thousands)	32.9	**27.0**	**31.3**
Applicants per 1,000 target population	1.6	**1.6**	**1.9**
Accepted applicants (thousands)	17.2	**15.7**	**17.2**
Applicant/acceptance ratio	1.9	**1.7**	**1.8**
Newly licensed MDs (thousands)	21.0	**17.6**	**21.0**
Percent FMGs of newly licensed MDs	23.1	**16.5**	**20.0**
Medical school income (billions of 1985 dollars)	11.0	**13.3**	**17.4**
Percent of medical school income from own revenues	41.0	**44.0**	**44.0**
Percent of all patient activities in teaching hospitals:			
Inpatient days	21.4	**22.4**	**23.3**
Outpatient visits	30.0	**28.9**	**29.4**
Research spending (billions of 1985 dollars)	0.19	**0.18**	**0.20**
Research concentration (percent research in top 20 medical schools)	50.0	**56.0**	**56.0**

Impact on Insurers

Insurers Face "Tough Choices"

Scenario I describes a long period of competitive struggle among insurance firms. After a brief period in the mid-1980s during which a wide variety of organizations--including providers, employers, and health care chains--tries its hand at health insurance, the system shakes out by the 1990s. It becomes very clear that some organizations are better than others in providing particular kinds of services. As described earlier, the key change in the structure of the health care system is the decline in use of fee-for-service and the growth in the contract and capitated sectors.

This structural shift is accompanied by a major competitive struggle over who pays. Although all major payers increase their dollar payments to the system, the share of all payments made by the public or government sector increases relative to that of private insurance and others (see table 52). This reflects the larger number of elderly covered by Medicare and the aggressive attitudes of businesses to the control of their benefit programs. Increasing copayments and the more rapid growth in employment in the service sector (where benefit coverage is more spotty) account for the relative decline. This is offset to some extent as more individuals and family groups seek some type of insurance to cover a larger portion of their liabilities that are not fully covered by government or employer programs.

Table 52
Source of Funds for Health Care (Percent of All Spending)

Year	Government	Private Insurance	Private Other
1970	37.0	22.5	40.5
1980	42.4	29.3	28.3
1985	41.1	31.4	27.5
1990	**41.7**	**31.1**	**27.2**
1995	**42.3**	**31.0**	**26.7**
2000	**42.8**	**30.9**	**26.3**

Within the private insurance market, the traditional insurers tend to hold onto much of the market that was threatened by newcomers in the early 1980s. The aggressive expansion of HMOs, hospital plans, and new corporate health groups was important for the early growth of the contract and capitated sector. But the traditional insurers respond in the late 1980s and early 1990s with contract and capitated programs of their own. The insurers' experience with administration and pricing serve them well in a market where cost control and efficient management are keys to success. By 2000, they increase their share of the capitated market to well over 50 percent and maintain a 75 percent share of the growing contract market (see table 53).

Table 53
Market Share of Traditional Insurers
(Percent of Each Market Held by Traditional Insurers)

Year	Contract Care	Capitated Care
1985	76	30
2000	**75**	**56**

The competitive marketplace favors those who can take advantage of economies of scale and those who have extensive local presence. This favors the very largest of the commercial insurers and the Blue Cross/Blue Shield Plans. In fact, just among commercial insurers the share of market held by the four largest firms goes up sharply in the 1990s, reversing a long-term decline during the era when there was little price competition (see table 54).

Table 54
Concentration Ratio among Commercial Insurers
(Percent of Commercial Market* Held by Four Largest Firms)

Year	Percent
1960	29.7
1985 (est.)	19.0
2000	**23.0**

*Excludes Blue Cross/Blue Shield

The struggle of the government to meet just the needs of those in existing benefit programs assures that the uninsured remain a problem.

The number and rate of uninsured drops slightly in the 1990s as a greater portion of the aging population moves under the protection of the Medicare system and through state-mandated risk pools or federally required extensions of private coverage. But, on the whole, public confusion about the uninsured remains high. The most vulnerable groups--the elderly and the very poor--have programs tailored to their needs and reduce the public's perception that something needs to be done now. Those without coverage are an odd lot: low-wage workers in small businesses, immigrants, recently divorced mothers, the young just moving out on their own, early retirees, the poor who can't find their way into the system. With no consensus on a systematic national health insurance plan, this mixed group of uninsured remain outside the system (see table 55).

Table 55
Uninsured Population

Year	Millions of People	Percent of Population
1985	35	15
2000	**32**	**12**

The government has its hands full meeting current benefit program needs. The growth in the number of elderly pushes total spending on Medicare up by some 60 percent (from $72 billion in 1985 to $116 billion in 2000, in 1985 dollars). Medicaid and other government spending also rises substantially but by smaller percentage amounts (Medicaid by 50 percent, from $42 billion in 1985 to $63 billion in 2000).

The movement toward more contract care and more capitated care does not come free. The net cost of health insurance--which includes the administrative costs of public and private sector insurance and profits flowing to for-profit organizations--rises sharply during this period. The costs of managing the more complex contracts is high as benefit administrators demand more information on the care administered, the costs of each element of that care, and measures of the quality of that care (see table 56). In addition, providers spend more administering, controlling their own costs, and developing data on the quality of care being provided.

Table 56
Net Cost of Insurance

Year	Percent of All Health Care Spending	Billions of 1985 Dollars
1970	3.7	7.5
1985	6.2	26.2
2000	**7.2**	**45.0**

Thus, the contract and capitated care sectors shake out to some extent. The large institutional players of the early 1980s--commercial insurers and the Blues--have carved out and defended their share of each of these sectors. The shares reflect the ability of large organizations to weather a long competitive struggle. The ones with dedication, capital reserves, and extensive local contacts survive. Certainly, there are some new players in the health insurance sector but not as many as the "hype" in the early 1980s had once suggested.

Insurers Under "Health and Wealth"

Under Scenario II, a plethora of hybrid health insurance forms emerge. The creation of gigantic vertically integrated "supermeds" stalls after the mid-1980s spasm of cost containment. Vertical integration does not work, because it places providers (who have an incentive to increase costs) under the same roof as insurers (who have an incentive to contain costs). This schizophrenia is aggravated by the rapid expansion of services during the 1990s. But managed care in its broadest sense is still a growing phenomenon. Traditional insurers--the Blues and commercials--are major players in the managed care business. They completely dominate the managed fee-for-service business, maintain three-quarters of the market as management intermediaries in contract care, and are responsible for over 60 percent in capitated care. Even in the fully integrated sector, the share of traditional insurers increases from 2 percent in 1985 to 15 percent in 2000. Overall, traditional insurers remain in the driver's seat in the reimbursement and financial management of health care.

Insurers do continue to exert cost containment pressures, but that function is no longer their main attraction to business or individuals. Instead, insurers compete on range, flexibility, and quality of services: claims processing speed and accuracy, maximum benefits per dollar in premiums, the ability to take over the utilization review that business finds too onerous, and the quality of their information on the relative cost effectiveness of new technologies. Insurers thus become guarantors of provider quality and consumer satisfaction.

To attain this vision of quality, horizontal integration occurs in the insurance market as well as among hospitals. Larger size permits higher expenditures on information systems and access to more patient data for pattern analysis and research. Increased size also provides insurers with the resources needed to deal with state-required mandated benefits and consumer-chosen cafeteria benefit plans. Large firms both can cover the broad markets and compete in the small high-cost niches. This consolidation leads to a higher level of concentration in the commercial insurance industry (see table 57).

Table 57
Concentration Ratio Among Commercial Insurers
(Percent of Commercial Market* Held by the Four Largest Firms)

Year	Percent
1970	28.3
1975	25.1
1980	22.8
1985 (est.)	19.0
1990	**20.0**
1995	**21.5**
2000	**23.0**

*Excludes Blue Cross/Blue Shield

The change in the concentration ratio (the share of the market held by the top four firms) is somewhat complicated by the issue of self-insurance, which will shrink as a share of the market largely because of the growth in managed care and the difficulties in separating risk-bearing from management. In any event, the concentration ratio will rise slightly by 2000, from 19 percent to 23 percent, reversing the historical downward trend. One reason is the spread of state-required mandated benefits (imposed on the grounds that everyone is entitled to certain types of coverage). These requirements make it harder for small firms to compete, since they have to offer full, and larger, product lines to group policy customers, even if some of the products are uneconomical. Cafeteria benefits plans have a similar effect.

These factors would drive the concentration ratio even higher but for the benign economic atmosphere that keeps even poor health care performers afloat. Many of the smaller players find very viable niches specializing in certain types of products, particularly capitated plans, in certain specific metropolitan areas. It has become fashionable in the industry to see giant insurers take on smaller insurers as subcontractors in these markets.

In insurance, as in care delivery, for-profit firms make a comeback in market share. Seeking predictable profit patterns, these insurers stress the continued shift of risk to the ultimate payer, the patient. Insurer profitability declines somewhat in the early 1990s, due to constant environmental change. Shifts in both federal and state program regulations, the imposition of mandated benefits, and the higher marketing and administration costs associated with specialized insurance products all diminish profitability. By the end of the century, however, profit rates are higher than in 1985. Some small insurers have been forced out of the market, increasing profits for those that remain, and the economy is performing well, which raises the return from invested premiums. Technological advances in claims processing (such as direct electronic data submission from providers) lower production costs.

Budget expansions and regulatory changes reduce the number of uninsured during the 1990s. A more affluent population is better able to insure itself and more willing to vote for increases in social spending. State-run risk pools extend coverage to previously uninsured groups. Congress, which extended group coverage in 1986 to people who would otherwise lose it due to divorce or layoffs, later extends retiree benefits even further. Another key factor underlying the reduction in uninsured is the maturing of the service economy. As the baby boom passes through the prime entrepreneurial age, the rate of new enterprise formation slows. Small businesses continue to grow in size, and a large proportion of them reaches a size threshold that allows them to buy group plans. Table 58 details the effects of these changes by the year 2000.

Table 58
Uninsured Population

	1985 (Estimated)	2000
Millions of People	35	16
Percent of Total Population	15	6

Government continues to play a major role in health care. As payer for the elderly and the poor, its role inevitably increases in the late 1980s and 1990s as these groups demand a greater number of services (see table 59).

Table 59
Public Sector Spending (Percent)

Year	Government Share of National Health Expenditures
1970	37.0
1975	42.5
1980	42.4
1985	41.1
1990	41.7
1995	42.0
2000	42.0

In terms of specific program expenditures, Medicare grows at an average annual rate of 4.5 percent, reflecting both the costs of intensity of use of services per recipient--what some pundits call the catastrophic effects of catastrophic insurance--and the growth in the number of recipients at about 1.4 percent per year.

Table 60 shows the marked increase in Medicaid funding at 3.6 percent per year, which reflects the layers and layers of state initiated "bandaids" that were put in place to help the underinsured and the medically indigent.

Table 60
Government Health Spending (Billions of 1985 Dollars)

	1985	2000
Medicare	72.3	140.2
Medicaid	41.8	71.2
Other	60.7	120.6
Total government spending on health care	174.8	332.0

Administering this complex hybrid system is expensive. Table 61 shows the net cost of insurance for 1985 and 2000. This includes both public and private costs of administration and the profit of private companies. Net cost rose sharply between 1984 and 1985, rising from 4.9 percent to 6.2 percent of the health care dollar; the rise was due to the impact of changing reimbursement systems as DRGs were imposed and assimilated. However, DRGs are not the last organizational innovation in the reimbursement system in the 1990s, with the result that transition and administration costs remain high. In addition, many new insurance products are diffused through the health care system: long-term care coverage, "boutique" products such as coverage for certain occupations, and so on. The spread of cafeteria plans and individualized "wellness" premium rebates virtually spell the end of traditional group contracts with their lower unit costs. The continuation of utilization and quality review under the roof of the insurers is another factor that will keep net cost high. It costs money to manage care. In short, the baroque health insurance market maintains net insurance cost at over 6 percent of total health care spending, nearly doubling it in real terms.

Table 61
Net Cost of Insurance

	1985		2000	
	Billions of 1985 Dollars	Percent of Total Health Care Spending	Billions of 1985 Dollars	Percent of Total Health Care Spending
Total	26.2	6.2	49.0	6.2
Private	20.4	4.8	34.0	4.3
Public	5.8	1.4	15.0	1.9
Federal	3.2	0.8	9.0	1.1
State/local	2.6	0.6	6.0	0.8

What Does It Mean?

The common characteristics between the two scenarios are important. The large traditional insurance firms do well after the threats of the 1980s. They continue to take advantage of the economies of scale they have as well as their ability to organize and manage information technology and to utilize sophisticated management, pricing experience, access to capital, and widespread local presence. The more effective management of insurance firms stops the trend to self-insure. Finally, the cost of administration remains high for both public and private insurers, taking a higher share of total health care dollars in the United States than in most other industrial countries.

The scenarios identify a few key uncertainties. Insurers could find that the key driver is cost containment or that the key driver is the push to uncover and develop market niches. The role of government could be very different, ranging from a policy governed by cost containment to one based on quality and expanded benefits. These uncertainties have profound effects on the roles that insurers will be required to play. Finally, the number of uninsured could vary dramatically, as well as the type of coverage granted to those currently uninsured if the extent of coverage was to expand significantly.

Table 62 (at the end of this chapter) and Appendix F show a summary of comparative insurer characteristics for both scenarios. (See Appendix B--Phase 3: Health Care Scenarios and Issues, for a description of the process used to generate issues.) Insurers face eight major issues:

1. New markets. The federal government is shifting more responsibilities to the states and through mandated coverage to the private sector. Both of these shifts are likely to slow the rapid growth in the public sector and may create attractive opportunities for private insurance. Included may be opportunities for insuring part-time workers, the uninsured and underinsured, individuals covered under Medicare and the Civilian Health and Medical Program of the Uniformed Services, and perhaps others. A major challenge will be the design of insurance products and assumption of risks that can lead to profitable ventures. Although privatization does open up new markets, many of these may not be attractive (for example, Medicare HMOs) or may pit insurers against large employers such as GM or Chrysler. It is likely that some innovative public/private plans can be structured such as those being considered by some states in waiving Medicaid "spend down" requirements if an individual has purchased a private long-term care policy.

2. Insurer/provider relationships. Insurers traditionally have worked closely with providers in establishing both standards and prices. Managed care will create a more adversarial role with providers and a call for a rethinking of positioning strategies among many insurance organizations. For example, insurers will need to structure contractual arrangements with providers specifying conditions for utilization reviews, second opinions, referrals, capitation arrangements, use of technology, and so forth. As a result, some of the saving of reduced utilization will be offset by the increased costs of management. In a real sense, insurers will be competing more directly with providers for a shrinking "cost containment" dollar. Managed care will not come cheaply.

3. Complexity of contracting. Insurers will find rapid shifts in the employee benefit market as competitive forces push to expand the range and flexibility of packages being offered. For example, the Blues will need to build contractual links with other players to be able to offer full-service benefit packages (coordinating life, health, disability, pensions, auto insurance) and effective benefit counseling to individual workers undergoing changes in personal or family needs. Insurers in general also will be increasingly

involved in new types of contracts with their traditional partners --the providers. The changing demands from both new and existing partners will substantially increase the complexity of insurance contracts in the future.

4. Paying for vulnerable groups. A number of high-risk or vulnerable groups, whose insurance needs are not being met in the current system, need special access to health care. The most obvious of these vulnerable populations are the uninsured and those in need of long-term care. As new high-risk groups emerge, like AIDS patients, the question arises as to whether coverage will be handled by the public or private sector. Those who contract AIDS and have to stop work will, in time, lose their employment insurance coverage. The increased financial burden of AIDS on those individuals and their families will likely stimulate government action to create special risk-pooling and financing arrangements for these groups. From the insurer's pespective, AIDS represents a tremendous potential for adverse selection in health insurance and, perhaps more significantly, in life insurance. With major high-risk or vulnerable groups, the key initiative must be taken by the public sector, though substantial opportunity for action by the private sector remains.

5. Quality and insurers. Quality will become of increasing concern to a sophisticated clientele as both educational levels and affluence rise and information becomes more easily accessible. Insurers will become a prime guarantor of quality. This fact will favor the large traditional insurance organizations, but it also will provide a unique opportunity for smaller firms to carve out profitable niches. It seems probable that insurers will also play a critical role in managing quality: ensuring that cost containment policies are not taken too far. They would use it as a means of managing malpractice risks and as a tool for marketing their products and affiliated providers. Insurers--and state governments--may take action on quality whether or not it will be palatable to providers. For example, it is likely that the increasing use of computerized databases, expert systems, and clinical algorithms will form the backbone of any quality assurance system. Key questions will arise on who has access to the databases, how such evidence will be used to intervene in cases of poor quality, and the extent to which detailed information of this type will be available to insurers, employers, or even patients and their lawyers.

6. Tax and antitrust policies. Government regulatory policy will have a big impact on insurers in two areas: tax and antitrust. In the need for budget funds, governments may impose new taxes on health insurance. This will slow the growth of such insurance

by shifting a greater burden of payment onto the individual, particularly those that receive "excessively generous benefits." Also, Blue Cross/Blue Shield could lose its nonprofit status entirely, and individual Blues plans could be forced to compete with each other. The effect of these changes could result in a radical restructuring of Blues plans in the form of state and regional consolidations. It is not clear whether these changes would have much impact on the competitive climate for health insurance more generally since the marginal effects of loss of tax exempt status and access to new sources of capital could be largely self-cancelling.

7. Ethical conflicts. In many cases, insurers will find themselves in the midst of conflicts where incentives diverge between cost and service, payer and patient, hospital and outpatient setting, technology and cost. Systematic ways of handling such conflicts need to be developed. For example, the courts, the medical profession, patients, their families, and their spiritual advisors could all play a role in deciding on questions of care for the terminally ill, the rights of patients to die, the questions of abortion, in-vitro and in-vivo fertilization, and so forth. The major policy question is: who has the right to decide? It is likely that there will be considerable variation between states on how such rights and responsibilities are distributed. Another key question revolves around the relative role of institutions--insurance companies, hospitals, medical associations, or universities--and the individuals who work within these institutions. To what degree are ethical choices to be made by individuals or the institutions they serve? For example, is it the responsibility of the hospital to develop an explicit policy on care for the terminally ill, or is it the responsibility of individual physicians and their patients? What are the legal and liability implications to insurers--as well as to others--of each alternative?

8. Cultural change among the Blues. Blue Cross/Blue Shield plans historically have had close cultural ties to hospitals and physicians. As competitive pressures build, it may become increasingly necessary for the Blues to develop an adversarial stance with providers. This change from facilitator of payment to manager of care will be difficult for all insurers, but particularly for the Blues. The close historical ties with providers may prove to be a benefit in marketing and product development, but the rules of the game are changing with three important implications for management style and strategic orientation. First, the modified tax status of Blues plans is a step closer to removing the Blues' unique image of a benevolent health insurer (benevolent in the minds of patients and providers) and placing them more firmly in the camp of commercial insurance. Second, in order to reinforce their "core" businesses, the Blues will come under increasing competitive pressure to enter other

lines of insurance business, such as life, disability, even auto insurance. A final question for Blues plans lies in the impact of these environmental changes on personnel. If a market reorientation of the Blues is under way, are the current management and staff appropriate for the new environment?

Table 62
Insurers: Comparative Summary of Scenarios

Indicator	1985	2000 I	2000 II
Market share of top four commercial insurers (percent)	19	23	23
Market share of traditional insurers in managed care:			
Contract (percent)	76	75	75
Capitated (percent)	30	56	60
Uninsured population (millions)	35	32	16
Uninsured population (percent)	15	12	6
Program administration and net cost of insurance (billions of 1985 dollars)	26.2	45.0	49.0
Government health spending (billions of 1985 dollars):	174.8	267.0	332.0
Medicare	72.3	116.0	140.2
Medicaid	41.8	63.0	71.2
Other (including R&D, construction, and public health)	60.7	88.0	120.6

Impact on Public Policy

Public Policy Concerns Under "Tough Choices"

AFFORDABILITY AND ACCESS

The cost of the elements of the health care system continues to rise but on a much more moderate basis than in the past. The cost of physician services on a per capita basis rises from $390 in 1985 to $407 (in 1985 dollars) in 2000. The cost of a day in the hospital as a percent of average weekly salaries also moderates in the 1990s (see table 63). The cost element that continues to rise rapidly is the cost of program administration and net cost of insurance. As cost controls become bureaucratized, the number of managers and administrators proliferate, and the share of all expenditures going to program administration and net cost of insurance rises from 3.7 percent in 1980 to 6.2 percent in 1985 to 7 percent in 2000.

Table 63
Hospital Costs (As a Percent of Average Weekly Earnings)

Year	Percent
1975	81.8
1980	104.3
1985	153.9
2000	**160.0**

The number of uninsured in the United States is reduced from 15 percent of the population to 12 percent. With the most vulnerable groups--the elderly and the very poor--covered by government programs tailored to their needs, it is difficult to mobilize public opinion on the issue of a national system of coverage. Many of those without coverage--low-wage workers in small businesses, recent immigrants, the recently divorced, the young moving out on their own--either pay for their care, do without, or utilize public hospitals and clinics. In fact, during the 1990s, about 5 percent of Americans continue to report on public surveys that they did not get medical care for financial reasons, virtually the same percentage that reported such a problem in the mid-1980s. In addition, health care institutions in the year 2000 report that their bill for uncompensated care remains at around 6 percent of gross hospital revenues, about where it was in 1985.

Because of the fairly strict reimbursement rules both by the government and by private insurers, access to the system is relatively cheap. In fact, the mean fee for a physician visit at $28 (in 1985 dollars) in 2000 is about the same that it was in 1985.

QUALITY

Quality in health care becomes a hotly debated issue in the 1990s with no clear consensus on a precise measure of performance. However, two measures that are mentioned often are the diffusion and appropriate utilization of technology and the satisfaction of people who use the health care system. Despite cost constraints, new proven technologies continue to diffuse rapidly. Figure 30 compares the diffusion rates of two proven technologies--CT scanners and cardiac catheterization--with one that represents high cost and high sophistication: organ transplantation. The former diffuse fairly rapidly, especially in the larger hospitals, as they prove their efficacy in well-defined circumstances, provide cheaper alternatives to more radical interventions, and as technology becomes somewhat cheaper and easier to use. Organ transplantation, on the other hand, remains a high-cost alternative with quotas on available donors and specialty teams and uncertain returns for institutions that commit themselves to forming such specialized teams.

The variation in the actual utilization of technology narrows substantially because of the effectiveness and widespread use of standardized information systems and the reimbursement controls established by the government and large private insurers. Table 64 compares the variation in various types of procedures per 10,000 Medicare enrollees in thirteen states or regions across the United States and finds that the range of variation has narrowed sharply for some common procedures.

Figure 30
Penetration of Technology
(Percent of U.S. Community Hospitals with Particular Facilities)

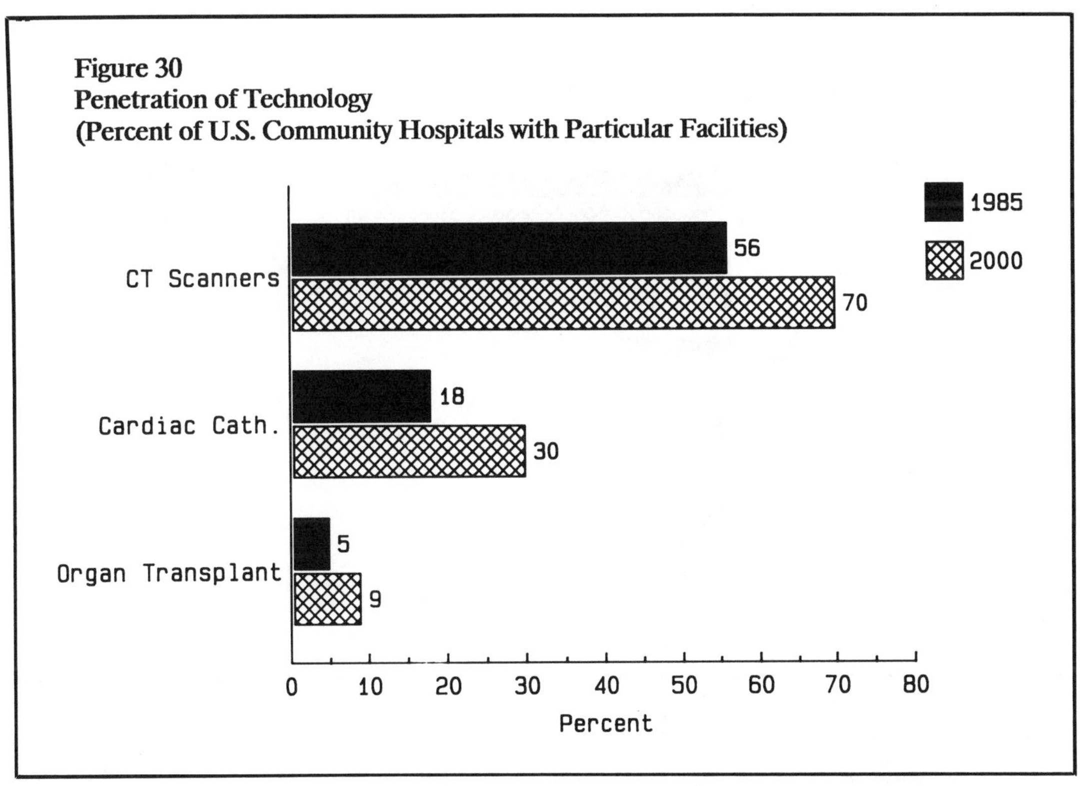

Table 64
Medical Care Variation
(Ratio of Highest Rate of Use to Lowest Rate of Use in 13 Sites)

Procedure	1981	2000
Coronary artery bypass	3.1	1.3
Total hip replacement	3.0	1.4
Diagnostic upper gastrointestinal endoscopy	1.6	1.2

Consumers' satisfaction with their own use of the health care system remains very high. Well over 80 percent of the public continues through the 1990s to express satisfaction with the health care services they have used (see figure 31). What does persist, however, is the markedly lower levels of consumer satisfaction for the poorest users of the health care system.

Figure 31
Consumer Satisfaction with Quality of Health Care

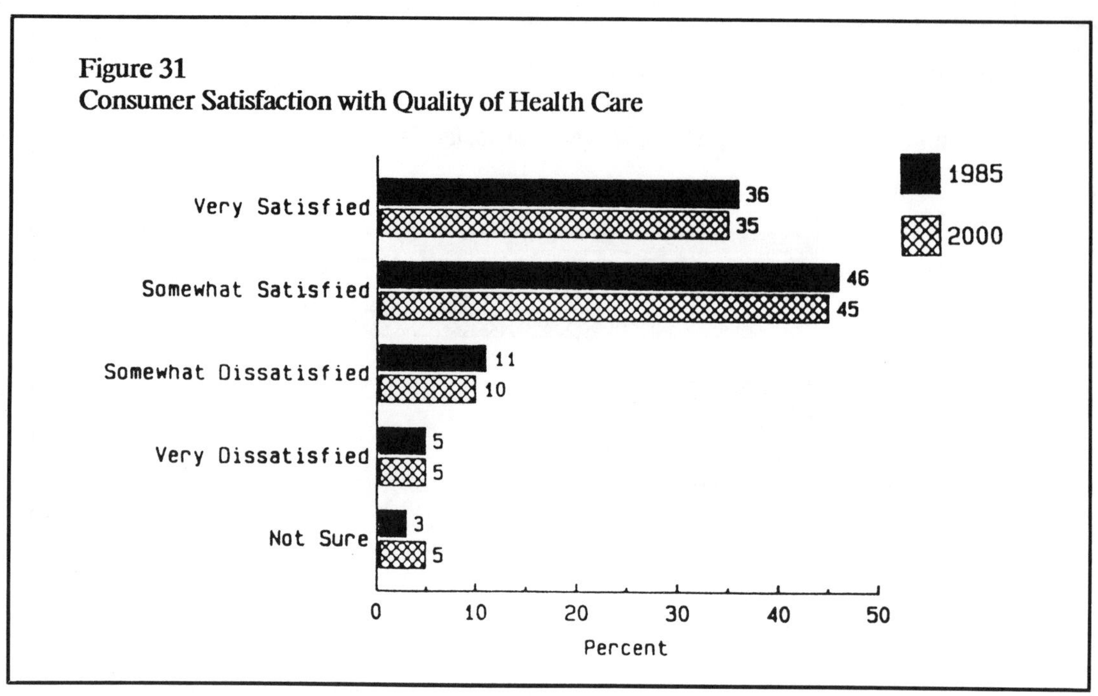

HEALTH STATUS

The links between health care and health status are not at all clear. Other societal factors like income, education, occupation, leisure habits, and eating patterns all make major contributions to changes. As measured by such traditional indicators as infant mortality, rates continue to fall, but progress is slow because many of the easy targets of improvement have been attained (see table 65).

Table 65
Infant Mortality Rates by Race (Deaths per 1,000 Live Births)

Year	Total	White	Black
1955	26.4	23.6	--
1965	24.7	21.5	41.7
1975	16.1	14.2	26.2
1984	10.8	9.4	18.4
2000	**7.9**	**7.0**	**12.0**

Americans spend more time and effort in taking care of themselves. A composite prevention index, established in the 1980s and reaching wide acceptability in the 1990s, measures the level of preventive behavior among the public that includes such factors as dieting, exercise, and risk behavior. Some improvement is noted, though progress is slow (see table 66).

Table 66
Prevention

Year	Prevention Index*
1985	63.2
2000	**69.0**

*An index ranging from 0 indicating that no one had taken any preventive steps to 100 where everyone interviewed had taken all reasonable preventive steps in 21 specific health promoting behaviors.

The uncertainty attached to the development of AIDS deserves a special mention. In this scenario, AIDS and the costs associated with the disease remain a prominent concern. Under the drive for cost effectiveness, the annual costs of treating a person diagnosed with AIDS comes to about $50,000 (in 1985 dollars). While we assume no "cure" emerges for AIDS, a routine for treatment has been established involving palliative drug therapies and treatment in clinics, outpatient settings, and hospices. These treatment centers are much less expensive than the hospital care that was common for AIDS patients in the late 1980s. Both public and private insurers, through their reimbursement policies, aggressively push for the development of a routine of care in outpatient or nonhospital settings and for the development of a variety of competing drug treatments. Support networks develop with the help of state and local funds and a variety of private and community groups. The total cost (in 1985 dollars) of AIDS to the health care system varies between $6 billion (if the rate of incidence reaches 125,000 in 2000) and $25 billion (if the rate of incidences reaches 500,000 in 2000). If all AIDS costs were counted as additional health care spending, the higher rate of incidence would add about 4% to total health care costs of $622 billion in 2000 to this scenario. This would raise the total spending on health care from 10.7 percent of GNP in 1985 to 11.1 percent of GNP in 2000. AIDS remains an important concern, but even with the higher rate of incidence, it does not deflect the drive for cost effectiveness.

In general, life expectancy continues to improve for Americans. Average expectancy rises from 74.7 years in 1985 to 77.6 years in 2000.

IMPACT ON EMPLOYMENT

The health care system continues to have an impact on the economy as a whole, though it plays a less dynamic role than it did in the 1960s, 1970s, and early 1980s--in both a positive and negative way. In the 1970s and early 1980s, health care contributed to the rapid escalation in inflation. Through the 1990s, health care costs are still rising faster than overall inflation but only by a moderate amount, and its inflationary impact on the rest of the economy is modest.

Health care is no longer a forceful driver of overall economic growth at either the national level or in various regional markets. The real value of health care expenditures, in fact, grows at the same rate as the economy as a whole. Yet, the job creation side of health care is important. Since health care remains a labor-intensive activity, employment in health care continues to grow faster than overall labor force growth, raising its share of total employment from 5.9 percent in 1985 to 7.0 percent in 2000 (see table 67).

Table 67
Health Care Employment (Percent)

Year	Health Care Employment	Total Employment	Share
1970	3.1	78.7	3.9
1985	6.3	107.2	5.9
2000	**9.1**	**130.2**	**7.0**

Public Policy Concerns Under "Health and Wealth"

SYSTEM AFFORDABILITY

Through the 1990s, the health care system continues to absorb a greater and greater share of national resources. What are the consumers, government, business, and philanthropists getting for their money? They clearly are getting more in volume terms, but are they getting more in value terms? One basic index of cost and affordability is the real per capita cost of physician services. This measure continues its apparently inexorable rise--as a result of more physicians, higher incomes, and increased intensity of services (see table 68).

Table 68
Physicians' Services--Cost per Capita (1985 Dollars)

Year	Physician Cost per Capita
1975	230
1985	390
2000	**546**

A second index of affordability is the cost of a day in the hospital --expressed as a share of average weekly earnings (see table 69).

Table 69
Hospital Costs (As a Percent of Average Weekly Earnings)

Year	Costs (Percent)
1975	81.8
1980	104.3
1985	153.9
2000	**185.0**

The average wage earner in 2000 has to work for more than nine days to pay the cost of one day in the hospital (up from just over five days in 1980). Again, this increase reflects the intensity of servicing in health care and the expense of new technologies.

A final measure of efficiency is the administrative cost of the system. The share of health care expenditures devoted to program administration and net cost of insurance rose rapidly in the early 1980s (see table 70). Part of this growth was the cyclical nature of the private insurance sector. But, to a large degree, the major jump in share was attributable to the administrative burden of cost management and marketing. This share does not increase appreciably by 2000, but the real costs increase by 80 percent in constant dollar terms. The share would have increased further if it were not for the productivity enhancing effects of information technology in helping the managers and marketers of health insurance.

Table 70
Program Administration and the Net Cost of Insurance (Percent)

Year	Share of National Health Expenditures
1965	3.8
1970	3.6
1975	3.3
1980	3.7
1985	6.2
2000	**6.2**

ACCESS

The uninsured and underinsured grow to be an enormous political problem in the late 1980s, and coverage is expanded incrementally through the late 1980s and early 1990s. Catastrophic coverage for Medicare is the first step. Then states begin a process of expanding Medicaid-like programs for certain low-income groups. In addition, in the wake of federal tax incentives, risk-pooling arrangements are mandated at the state level that bring into the system employees of small business and self-employed individuals who are willing and able to pay the true cost of group insurance. Many states also have introduced special insurance funds for AIDS victims. As a result, the number of Americans who are not covered by health insurance drops from 35 million in 1985 to 16 million in 2000. This residual group of uninsured is predominantly young, single, and healthy, and public policy concerns about the uninsured wane as it is realized that this group neither needs nor wants health insurance. However, if the uninsured really get into trouble--through accidents or other trauma--they do receive care on a charitable basis, usually at public hospitals. The bill for uncompensated care, however, is greatly reduced from almost 6 percent of gross hospital revenues in 1985 to 3 percent in 2000.

Although coverage has expanded, this does not mean the system is without access problems. The average cost of a physician visit for an established patient increases steadily in real terms at about 1.2 percent per year (see table 71). Since physician visits in most plans are subject to copayments and deductibles, these increases are somewhat onerous for certain heavy users of services.

Table 71
Mean Fee for a Physician Visit (1985 Dollars for an Established Patient)

Year	Fee
1974	23.9
1985	27.8
2000	**33.3**

The U.S. health care system continues to have a healthy appetite for technology. Technologies are adopted and diffused, both complex, expensive "halfway" technologies and low-cost "decisive" technologies. As an index of this availability, figure 32 shows the percentage of U.S. community hospitals offering three specific technologies.

Figure 32
Penetration of Technology
(Percent of U.S. Community Hospitals with Particular Facilities)

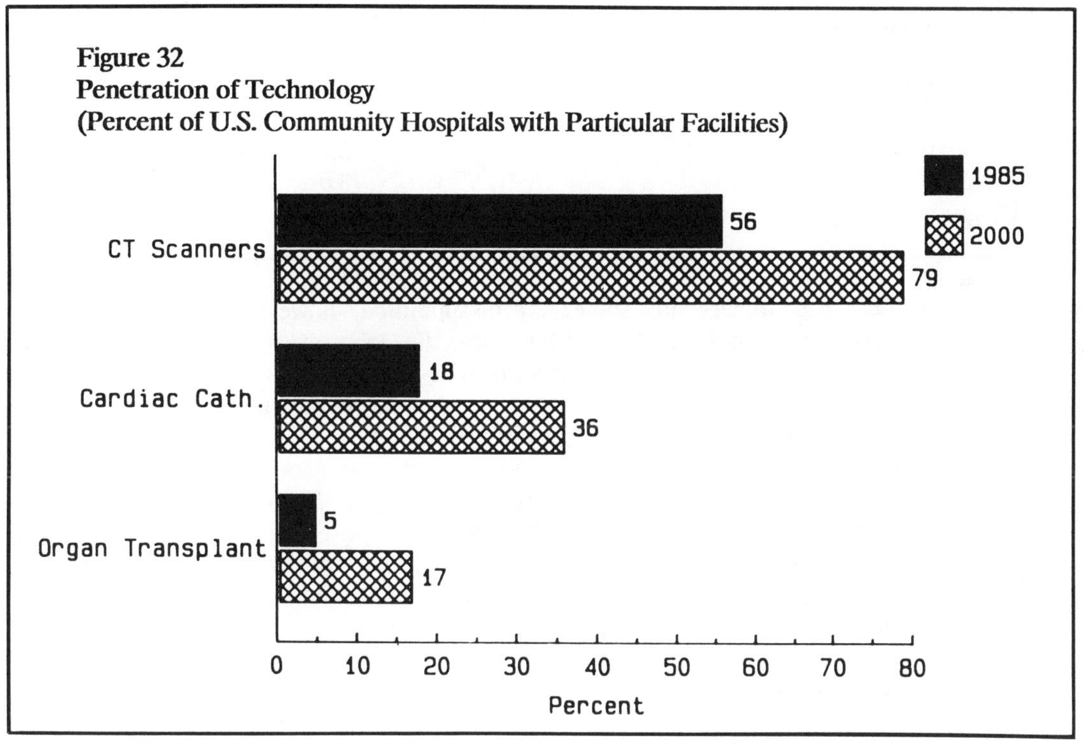

Certain technologies such as organ transplants are concentrated in large hospitals that have sophisticated support staffs and technologies and a high volume of patients. But other apparently expensive technologies are not so heavily centralized; indeed, some wiseacre notes in 2000 that there are more CT scanners than 7-11 stores.

QUALITY

During the 1990s, tremendous research efforts are made in defining and measuring health care quality. Despite the wealth of research findings, no clear consensus exists on the measures. Providers tend to favor process measures; economists and public health officials favor health status measures; and consumers use more subjective measures such as patient relations as well as perceptions of medical staff competence and knowledge. The research effort on quality has shown up in one key area: the so-called medical variation statistics. For example, a study in the mid-1980s reporting on 1981 data was updated in 2000 by the same researchers. They find that the variation in the rate of procedures per 10,000 enrollees in thirteen geographic sites across the United States has dropped considerably by 2000 (see table 72).

Table 72
Medical Care Variation
(Ratio of Highest Rate of Use to Lowest Rate of Use in 13 Sites)

Procedure	1981	2000
Coronary artery bypass	3.1	2.5
Total hip replacement	3.0	2.5
Diagnostic upper gastrointestinal endoscopy	1.6	1.5

Researchers are somewhat disappointed, however, that the drop in variation is not greater: they cite the lack of success in establishing medical consensus on clinical algorithms, the role of the consumer/patient in demanding certain procedures, and the continued variation in the practice settings and missions of the provider organizations.

Nevertheless, consumers--even some from lower income levels--are quite satisfied with health care services (see figure 33). Health is a consumer-driven industry in the 1990s, and most consumers do not object to paying more for services they feel they have some sovereignty in selecting. Nevertheless, a large group of Americans think changes are needed, particularly the young Americans who feel they are paying excessively high taxes and insurance costs to support this elaborate system with the prospect of paying even more when the baby boom reaches retirement.

Figure 33
Consumer Satisfaction with Quality of Health Care

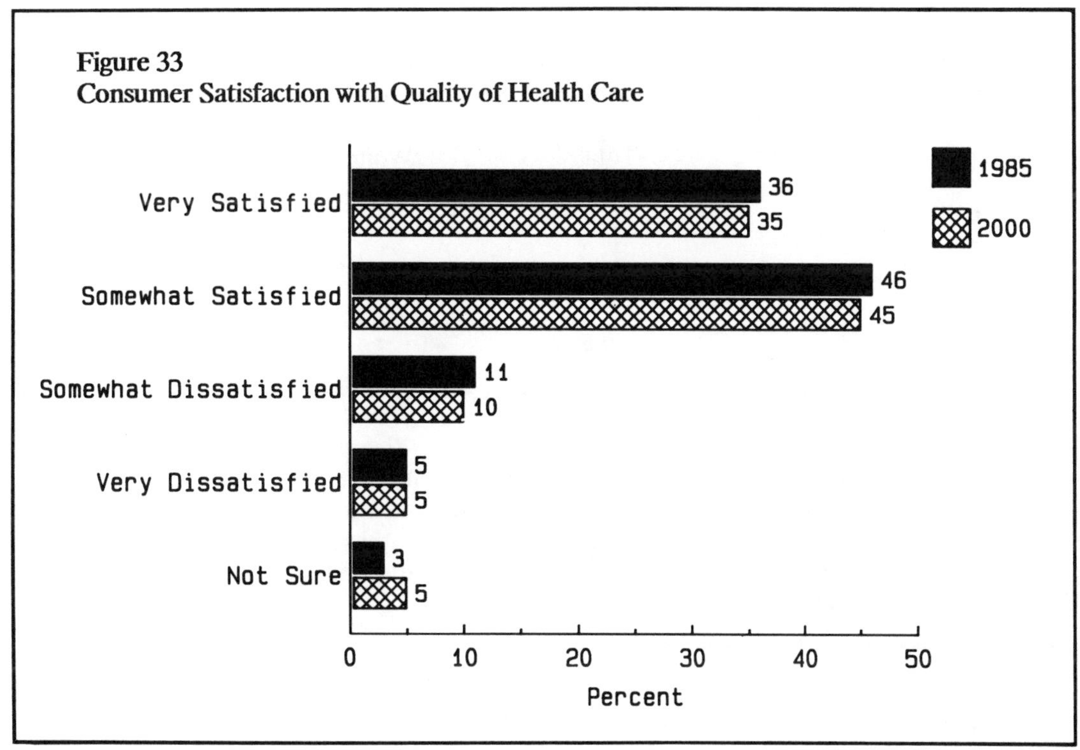

HEALTH STATUS

The links between expanded health care services and improvements in health status have never been very clear. The respective contribution to health status of such diverse variables as higher income and coronary surgery techniques continue to be difficult to weigh. Whatever the reason, traditional indicators of health status continue to improve. For example, infant mortality rates continue to drop for both whites and blacks (see table 73), but progress is slower than expected because of the lack of decline in the share of births that are defined as low birth weight. These high-risk births continue to be asymmetrically concentrated in the more vulnerable groups in society, and the programs to reach these groups have not been a high priority. It is important to note that a rising tide does lift all boats, and public health expenditures do increase in real terms; however, as we discuss below, the number one public health priority in the 1990s is the AIDS epidemic, which consumes an ever-increasing share of public health budgets, leaving other programs relatively less well off.

Table 73
Infant Mortality Rates by Race (Deaths per 1,000 Live Births)

Year	Total	White	Black
1955	26.4	23.6	--
1965	24.7	21.5	41.7
1975	16.1	14.2	26.2
1984	10.8	9.4	18.4
2000	**7.9**	**7.0**	**12.0**

Prevention is not the monopoly of the public health system: many Americans are taking better care of themselves. A composite prevention index is established in the 1980s that measures the level of preventive behavior among the public. Changes in this index show that steady, if not spectacular, progress is made toward good preventive behavior (see table 74).

Table 74
Prevention

Year	Prevention Index*
1985	63.2
2000	**72.0**

*An index ranging from 0 indicating that no one had taken any preventive steps to 100 where everyone interviewed had taken all reasonable preventive steps in 21 specific health promoting behaviors.

The major progress in the index comes from increased seat belt use, accident prevention, and moderation in smoking and alcohol consumption. Diet and exercise do not improve as much as once hoped, because, despite the fitness-conscious members of the baby boom, an entire generation of fast-food children find it hard to kick the habit.

Americans are living longer. Average life expectancy rises from 74.7 years to 78 years by 2000 (75 for men and 81 for women), and over 100,000 Americans are honorary members of ACE (Americans for Centigenerian Equity). Average life expectancy would be even higher if it were not for the specter of AIDS deaths over the mortality statistics.

AIDS is still the number one public health priority in America. Progress in prevention and increased awareness of the disease among the baby boom help slow the progression of the disease in the 1990s. However, a large number of people infected with the virus in the 1980s do not develop the disease until well into the 1990s, and, consequently, the economic and social burden of new AIDS cases continues to increase.

Progress has been made in palliative care that enables the medical system to help patients through acute bouts of illness. But, although these expensive drug regimens are reasonably effective, they are not a cure. Progress in developing a vaccine takes much longer than expected, and, by the mid-1990s, a number of vaccines are awaiting regulatory approval. The preferred treatment of AIDS involves a whole range of acute, chronic, rehabilitative, hospice, and preventive services as new research yields an increasing set of medical and social interventions.

The cost of AIDS treatment has escalated as new treatment modalities are developed and added: by the late 1990s, each new case incurs a direct health cost of $75,000 per annum (in constant 1985 dollars). Given that the estimated range of new AIDS cases per annum by 2000 is between 125,000 and 500,000, this translates into a total direct health care cost of AIDS of between $9.4 billion and $37.5 billion (in constant 1985 dollars). In a $6.2 trillion economy, the direct health costs of AIDS would range from 0.15 percent to 0.61 percent of GNP. In the extreme case, health care spending would rise from 12.7 percent of GNP to 13.3 percent of GNP.

IMPACT ON EMPLOYMENT

In the 1990s, health care supplants the defense industry as the backbone of advanced industrial economies. In the United States, health care is a major contributor to growth in employment and is a major target for new technology. However, the increased investment in human capital in health care is not simply an extrapolation of the rapid rates of growth of the 1960s and 1970s. Health care in the 1990s is still very labor intensive when compared to the steel industry, but it is much less labor intensive than in the 1970s. The increasing demands and constrained resources of the 1980s force health care institutions to invest more heavily in capital --particularly information technology. As a result, the annual average rate of growth in health care employment is 3.8 percent, even though the health care sector is growing at a real rate of 4.2 percent per annum from 1985 to 2000 (see table 75).

Table 75
Health Care Employment

Year	Health Care Employment (Millions)	Total Employment (Millions)	Share (Percent)
1970	3.1	78.7	3.9
1985	6.3	107.2	5.9
2000	**10.7**	**133.0**	**8.0**

Health care plays a central role in local and even regional economies. In older industrial cities, health care is by far the biggest employer; and in many of the less dynamic regions of the country, health care is the bright light on the employment scene. A key reason, of course, is that health care delivery remains relatively immune to international competition. However, the term "relatively" should be stressed because the United States in the 1990s has considerable trade in health care delivery. It exports hospital and health care management expertise to other countries and exports esoteric surgical procedures to rich foreign nationals. But many Americans living near the Canadian border are buying health care from their northern neighbors. The disparity in costs is so large that U.S. insurance companies are willing to pay air fare and hotel expenses to Canada as part of a block rate for certain elective surgical procedures.

What Does It Mean?

The scenarios outline two possible worlds of public policy. Some of the trends described are common to both of the scenarios: quality becomes a major public policy focus in both scenarios but for different reasons; ethical and economic choices surrounding the use of technology are difficult in both scenarios; health status and prevention continue to improve in both scenarios albeit at slightly different rates; and AIDS casts a frightening shadow over any scenario.

There are, however, key uncertainties in terms of the policy choices that will be made and the effects that they will have. A key uncertainty lies in access to health care for vulnerable groups--the uninsured, the elderly in long-term care, mothers and children, and those with AIDS. The responses vary from only modest improvement in access at the margin to incremental gains in programs that, in total, markedly improve access to care. There is also considerable uncertainty in other dimensions of public policy: tort reform and the malpractice question; attitudes toward health care as a source of employment; and consumer choice and involvement in health care. Table 76 (at the end of this chapter) and Appendix F show a summary of public policy indicators for both scenarios.

These key trends and uncertainties serve as the backdrop of public policymaking in health care through the balance of the century. The policy debate will likely center on eleven key issues. (See Appendix B--Phase 3: Health Care Scenarios and Issues, and Phase 4: Public Policy Issues, for a description of the processes used to generate issues.) All of these are high on the agenda today and will continue to be important in the next decade, in either scenario:

1. <u>Controlling costs</u>. No clear policy option has yet emerged as a winning solution to health care cost containment. In the course of this study, participants have raised and debated the merits of many policies to contain costs ranging from increased competition and personal accountability in the consumption of health care services to National Health Insurance. What is clear is that no national consensus exists on how to contain costs and, indeed, on whether to contain costs. The policy debate on controlling health costs is not over--it has been high on the agenda for the past fifteen years, and it will still be a high public policy priority in the future.

2. <u>The uninsured</u>. By the mid-1980s, approximately 15 percent of the population, or some 35 million individuals, do not have health insurance of any kind. In addition, a substantial proportion of the population, perhaps a further 20 percent, has only minimal coverage that is insufficient to allow them full access to the health care system. The key groups left out of the system are those working in low-paid service sector jobs, often in small companies; those in temporary or part-time work; and the dependents of these employees. The key policy questions are: who will pay for these groups, what is an acceptable minimum standard of care, and what should be the health care delivery system for these groups? The array of likely policy choices seems to be limited to mandating benefit coverage in small business, expanding Medicaid through changes in eligibility requirements, establishing state risk pools, and expanding direct financing to public institutions such as county hospitals that carry the weight of delivering care to the uninsured. Political pressures to expand access are likely to increase and will be driven by the increasing visibility of the uninsured, underinsured, and other high-risk groups such as AIDS victims.

3. <u>Long-term care</u>. The inevitable growth in the number of people over 65 and in particular those over 75 and 85 presents a major policy problem for the 1990s and beyond. The financial burden of long-term care could conceivably rise from 9 percent of health

costs to more than 15 percent by 2000. The critical policy questions now and in the future are: who pays and who provides the care? Individual households and families will continue to bear the greatest burden of long-term care--either through family support or through the accumulated assets of the elderly themselves. Private insurance plans and medical IRAs are likely to act more as a supplement than as a replacement to the family supported system. Medicaid, which, by default rather than design, currently funds almost half of institutional long-term care, could not absorb the anticipated costs of an aging population. Any other publicly funded program of institutional care for the elderly would seem unlikely unless government's financial position goes through a dramatic recovery in the 1990s. Considerable research is required to find innovative and inexpensive methods to finance and deliver long-term care that do not involve institutionalization.

4. Mother and child. Many public policy issues are multidimensional and can be resolved only through a variety of programs developed by different agencies. A key issue that is likely to gain prominence in the 1990s is the plight of disadvantaged mothers and their young children. As the proportion of children born into poverty has increased over the past decade, increasing attention is being drawn to the lack of prenatal maternal health care and the inadequacy of educational, preventive health, and social initiatives aimed at addressing the problems of teenage pregnancy, particularly among minority women. Although closely related to the wider problem of the uninsured, the issue of mother and child will require special attention in the 1990s.

5. AIDS. Not only is AIDS a major driver of change, but it has become increasingly clear that AIDS will be an enormously important policy issue in the 1990s. By the end of 1987, almost 50,000 Americans had contracted the disease, with more than 20,000 having died. An estimated 1 to 1.5 million people are infected with the virus. The AIDS issue involves broad societal choices about public health education, testing and reporting, and civil rights questions on housing, employment, and access to welfare and insurance. The health care system itself faces enormously difficult public policy challenges over who pays for care; where care will be provided; the role of the volunteer sector; the impact on attracting and compensating physicians and other health personnel; and coping with the extreme pressures on providers, insurers, and payers in the AIDS hot spots.

6. Quality in a competitive environment. In any scenario, quality will likely emerge as a critical issue. Whether it is driven by the need to ensure that quality doesn't suffer from cost contain-

ment or by the needs of providers, managed care organizations and insurers trying to market services on quality lines, the focus on quality is likely to intensify. The key questions revolve around measuring and managing quality and determining the role that various actors will play in these activities: state and federal governments, payers, insurers, the professions, and the courts. The availability of computer generated databases, the increased flow of information between provider and payers, and the increasingly competitive environment will intensify the scrutiny of the practice of medicine and erode the autonomy of the profession.

7. Health manpower. While the total number of people working in the health care field will continue to increase, needs will change over time. The move of more care to the outpatient setting will reduce the relative size of the hospital sector and change the composition of both patient care and support personnel. The shift to new types of outpatient technologies will affect the technical composition of the labor force. The growth of managed care will increase the role and influence of professional managers who will challenge the traditional supremacy of MDs in the field. Further, the financially strapped government will be more hesitant to provide large subsidies to training, and many of the implicit subsidies for training within the current reimbursement system will be phased out. In turn, as more physician training is self-financed through loans, the power of large organized medical practices will grow since they can offer financial security (and debt repayment) for young physicians.

8. Health R&D. Financing changes will affect the flow of funds into medical research. Tighter reimbursement rules will cut the implicit subsidies for academic medical centers. More concentration of research in the top academic research centers will raise the cost of both doing the research and getting regulatory approval. The growing cost of research will channel an increasing portion of both private and public funds into a few areas that draw wide publicity and promise great rewards. Research agendas will be reshaped so that research is driven by targeted customer needs rather than by the laboratory.

9. Redeploying capital. New competitive forces will bring important changes to the health care infrastructure of buildings and equipment. There will be some decline in the use of hospitals, especially smaller hospitals in nonmetropolitan areas. But there will be significant growth in outpatient facilities. The greater reliance on market forces will push many practitioners to seek locations convenient to key customers or to have available the latest technologies. This will produce a large need for a new flow of capital, but it

will be a capital flow responsive to market opportunities rather than the simple rule of increased access to the system which dominated government support in the 1960s and 1970s. The high cost of redeployment with the expected wide swings in interest rates will be a hardship for providers who do not have an assured income stream and ready access to financial markets.

10. Tort liability. The better educated, more sophisticated U.S. society wants to minimize its own risks in a complex world. The health care field is a growing target for lawsuits and litigation, and escalating insurance premiums will remain a problem. An even greater impact will come as potential liability affects the setting of practice standards. In fact, the ability to control practice patterns is likely to favor large, professionally managed practice groups because they can establish standardized procedures or policies that minimize exposure to risk.

11. Ethics. The institutional changes in the health care system will make some ethical choices more difficult. Doctors will be at the center. On the one hand, they will be trained to utilize a growing range of sophisticated technologies that relatively well-educated patients will be asking for; on the other hand, many of them will be working in institutional settings that use economic guidelines as to who gets what treatment in any particular situation. Further, other subtle conflicts will arise as physicians dispense drugs that they prescribe and administer more of their own diagnostic tests. Other conflicts will emerge as biomedical researchers in academic settings assume more important roles in biotechnology firms.

Table 76
Public Policy: Comparative Summary of Scenarios

Indicator	1985	2000 I	2000 II
Physician services per capita (1985 dollars)	390	407	546
Mean fee per physician visit (1985 dollars)	28	28	33.3
Hospital costs (percent of average weekly earnings)	153.9	160	185
Share of health expenditures to program administration and net cost of insurance (percent)	6.2	7.0	6.2
Penetration of technology (percent of U.S. community hospitals):			
CT scanners	56	70	79
Cardiac catheterization	18	30	36
Organ transplant	5	9	17
Medical care variation (highest/lowest in 13 sites):			
Coronary artery bypass	3.1 (1981)	1.3	2.5
Total hip replacement	3.0 (1981)	1.4	2.5
Diagnostic upper GI	1.6 (1981)	1.2	1.5
Consumer satisfaction with health care (percent very/somewhat satisfied)	72	70	70
Infant mortality rates	10.8 (1984)	7.9	7.9
Prevention index*	63.2	69	72
Health care employment (millions)	6.3	9.1	10.7

*An index ranging from 0 indicating that no one had taken any preventive steps to 100 where everyone interviewed had taken all reasonable preventive steps in 21 specific health promotion behaviors.

Appendix A

Study Participants

EXPERTS: ENVIRONMENTAL SCENARIOS

Bernard Anderson, Wharton Center for Applied Research, Philadelphia, PA
Clyde Behney, Health Program Manager, Office of Technology Assessment, Washington, DC
Theodore Cooper, M.D., Vice Chairman, Upjohn Company, Kalamazoo, MI
John Dunlop, Lamont University Professor, Harvard University, Cambridge, MA
Martin Feldstein, National Bureau of Economic Research, Cambridge MA
Victor Fuchs, Professor, Department of Economics, Stanford University, Stanford, CA
Eli Ginzberg, Director, Conservation of Human Resources, Columbia University, New York, NY
Alfred Kahn, Department of Economics, Cornell University, Ithaca, NY
Donald Kennedy, President, Stanford University, Stanford, CA
Charles Kindleberger, Professor, Economics Department, Massachusetts Institute of Technology, Cambridge, MA
Joshua Lederberg, M.D., Office of the President, Rockefeller University, New York, NY
Eppie Lederer (Ann Landers), Columnist, Chicago Sun Times, Chicago, IL
Seymour Lipset, Professor of Political Science, Stanford University, Stanford, CA
Paul Marks, M.D., President and Chief Executive Officer, Memorial Sloan-Kettering Cancer Center, New York, NY
Barbara J. McNeil, M.D., Brigham and Women's Hospital, Boston, MA
Walter L. Robb, Senior Vice President and Group Executive, General Electric Medical Systems Group, Milwaukee, WI
F. David Rollo, M.D., Senior Vice President, Medical Affairs, Humana, Inc., Louisville, KY
Walter A. Rosenblith, Massachusetts Institute of Technology, Cambridge, MA
Paul Samuelson, Professor, Economics Department, Massachusetts Institute of Technology, Cambridge, MA
Charles Schultze, Brookings Institution, Washington, DC
Humphrey Taylor, President, Louis Harris and Associates, New York, NY

PANELISTS: HEALTH CARE SCENARIOS AND ISSUES

Bruce E. Balfe, Vice President, Health Policy Management, American Medical Association, Chicago, IL
H. Thomas Ballantine, M.D., private practitioner, Boston, MA
Richard F. Corlin, M.D., private practitioner, Santa Monica, CA
John C. Gaffney, Director, Office of Policy Analysis and Planning, American Medical Association, Chicago, IL
William D. Marder, Director, Department of Health Resource Analysis, American Medical Association, Chicago, IL
James F. Rodgers, Director, Center for Health Policy Research, American Medical Association, Chicago, IL
C. Burns Roehrig, M.D., private practitioner, Boston, MA
Dale A. Rublee, Policy Analyst, Department of Health System Analysis, Center for Health Policy Research, American Medical Association, Chicago, IL
John Kimball Scott, M.D., private practitioner, Madison, WI
Frank B. Walker II, M.D., private practitioner, Grosse Pointe Farms, MI
Ross H. Weaver, Director, Office of Technology Management, American Medical Association, Chicago, IL
Andrew D. Weinberg, M.D., private practitioner, Branford, CT

Christian J. Anton, Senior Vice President, St. Alphonsus Regional Medical Center, Boise, ID
Henry Bachofer, Director, Division of Health Policy and Hospital Finance, American Hospital Association, Chicago, IL
Gary L. Fletcher, Chief Executive Officer, Central Montana Hospitals, Lewistown, MT
Roland E. Kohr, President, Bloomington Hospitals, Bloomington, IN
Wayne Lerner, Vice President, Administration, Rush-Presbyterian-St. Lukes Medical Center, Chicago, IL
John M. Lowe, Vice President, Hospital Research and Educational Trust, Chicago, IL
Joseph R. Martin, Director, Division of Health Economic Studies and Hospital Data Center, American Hospital Association, Chicago, IL
Larry L. Mathis, President and Chief Executive Officer, Methodist Hospital, Houston, TX
Bruce McPherson, President, Hospital Research and Educational Trust, Chicago, IL
Ross Mullner, Director, Hospital Research Center, American Hospital Association, Chicago, IL
Mitchell T. Rabkin, M.D., President, Beth Israel Hospital, Boston, MA
C. Thomas Smith, President, Yale New Haven Hospital, New Haven, CT
Gordon M. Sprenger, President, Abbott Northwestern Hospital, Minneapolis, MN
Edwin Tuller, Vice President, Division of Corporate Planning, American Hospital Association, Chicago, IL

Ronald C. Wacker, Director, Division of Hospital Planning, Capital Finance, and Special Studies, American Hospital Association, Chicago, IL

Victor Crown, Special Assistant to the Dean, University of Pennsylvania School of Medicine, Philadelphia, PA
Sheldon S. King, President, Stanford University Hospital, Stanford, CA
Richard M. Knapp, Director, Department of Teaching Hospitals, Association of American Medical Colleges, Washington, DC
Richard L. O'Brien, M.D., Dean and Vice President for Health Services, Creighton University School of Medicine, Omaha, NE
Robert G. Petersdorf, M.D., President, Association of American Medical Colleges, Washington, DC
Edward J. Stemmler, M.D., Dean, University of Pennsylvania School of Medicine, Philadelphia, PA
Virginia Weldon, M.D., Deputy Vice Chancellor for Medical Affairs, Washington University Medical School, St. Louis, MO

John Brouse, Senior Vice President, Private Business, Pennsylvania Blue Shield, Camp Hill, PA
Donald R. Cohodes, Executive Director, Policy, Blue Cross and Blue Shield Association, Chicago, IL
Dexter Coolidge, Executive Director, Business Strategy Services, Blue Cross and Blue Shield Association, Chicago, IL
Michael Graves, Senior Vice President, Group Products, Blue Cross of Western Pennsylvania, Pittsburgh, PA
Arthur E. Hall, Jr., Vice President, Strategic Planning, Community Mutual Insurance Company, Cincinnati, OH
Suzanne Mulstein, Senior Consultant, Policy, Blue Cross and Blue Shield Association, Chicago, IL
Michael Walsh, Corporate Vice President, Corporate Planning and Strategies, Empire Blue Cross and Blue Shield, New York, NY

PUBLIC POLICY PANELISTS: PUBLIC POLICY ISSUES

John Brademus, President, New York University, New York, NY
John T. Dunlop, Lamont University Professor, Harvard University, Cambridge, MA
Eli Ginzberg, Director, Conservation of Human Resources, Columbia University, New York, NY
Robert M. Heyssel, M.D., President, Johns Hopkins Hospital, Baltimore, MD
Walter J. McNerney, Professor of Health Policy, J. L. Kellogg Graduate School of Management, Northwestern University, Evanston, IL
Cyrus Vance, Simpson, Thacher & Bartlett, New York, NY

OTHER EXPERTS

Theodore Bernstein, Director of ILGWU Benefit Fund, International Ladies Garment Workers Union, New York, NY
William Ehrich, Manager of Medical and Health Care Benefits, IBM Corporation, Armonk, NY
Robert Evans, Professor, Department of Economics, University of British Columbia, Vancouver, B.C., Canada
Richard Finucane, M.D., Vice President and Corporate Medical Director, General Foods, White Plains, NY
George A. Fromme, Division Manager, Benefit Planning and Analysis, AT&T, New York, NY
John Kitteridge, Executive Vice President, Prudential Insurance, Newark, NJ
Philip R. Lee, M.D., Professor of Social Medicine, Institute for Health Policy Studies, University of California at San Francisco, San Francisco, CA
Steven Markman, Research Associate, Human Resources Program Group, The Conference Board, New York, NY
Thomas McVeigh, Director, Personnel Benefits, CBS, Inc., New York, NY
Robert Patricelli, Vice President, CIGNA Corporation, Bloomfield, CT
Stanley J. Reiser, M.D., Griff T. Ross Professor of Humanities and Technology in Health Care, University of Texas Health Science Center at Houston, Houston, TX

Appendix B

Study Methodology

INTRODUCTION

Our general objective was to develop alternative and comprehensive pictures of the future health care system. Such pictures should be suitable for use by major health care actors in identifying and understanding key issues and choices. Because of the incomplete understanding of driving forces, structural interrelationships, and choices that may be made by various actors--as well as the possible occurrence of unexpected and unanticipated developments--our aim was clearly not to make "point forecasts" nor to use econometric models that reflect primarily historical relationships.

SCENARIOS

Our approach relied heavily on the integrated judgments of a group of carefully selected individuals. To summarize and portray the perceptions of the group, we have selected a particular vehicle--the scenario form. Scenarios are internally consistent descriptions of alternative and plausible futures. They may be used for a variety of purposes, but increasingly they are used to summarize alternative assumptions about the future. In this instance, scenarios are used to portray the uncertainty and to describe alternative paths along which the health care environment may evolve. The aim is to highlight issues or choices that are likely to be faced by the principal health care stakeholders and the larger society.

Scenarios provide a powerful medium for portraying the inherent uncertainties in health care. To do so, of course, at least two scenarios are required to span the principal domain over which variations of variables are expected. At times, three or four scenarios may be used, but the addition of each scenario increases the complexity and increases the likelihood that attention will focus on a particular scenario falling in the "mid" range. For example, with three scenarios the tendency is to pick the "center" scenario and to ignore the side ones. In the final analysis, the choice of the number and the "positioning" of scenarios is dictated by the range of perceptions contained in the elicited information, the analysis of this information, the uses to which the scenarios are to be put, and the judgment of the scenario writers. We chose to portray the future health care environment in the form of two plausible and distinct scenarios.

STUDY PROCESS

The overall study process is shown in figure B-1. The four major phases are described below.

Phase 1: Descriptors and Factors (Figure B-2)

Our starting point was to identify a set of key descriptors of the health care system. A descriptor is a characteristic of the health care system--preferably quantitative--that tells us something about the "state" of the system. Clearly, different descriptors are of primary interest to different players. On a societal level, such descriptors include information on cost, access, quality, and health status. For specific groups such as physicians, hospitals, academic medical centers, and insurers, the list may include: physician income, hospital admissions, the number of academic medical centers, and percent enrollment in capitation-based systems. Through a series of in-depth interviews and/or workshops,* we identified well over 100 candidate descriptors. These were distilled to an essential set of about forty that provided the focus for the study (see summary tables, and Chapters 5 through 8 for the final list used).

At this point, the descriptor set was used as a point of departure to identify those factors in the environment external to health care that could affect these descriptors. We conducted another set of interviews and workshops to identify those factors. Specific items fell into the following major categories: the state of the economy, demography, households/lifestyles, attitudes, role of government, and technology (the full list is shown in table B-1). Equally as important as the specific factors identified was the rationale or logic that connected particular health care system descriptors to particular external factors. For example, hospital admissions as influenced by changes in the proportion of the aged, the cost of health care as affected by changing attitudes toward dying, the number of academic medical centers as influenced by pressures of growing budget deficits, and so forth.

*For a description of specific techniques used, see Roy Amara and Andrew Lipinski, *Business Planning for an Uncertain Future,* Elmsford, New York: Pergamon Press, 1983, Chapter 4, pp. 49-51.

Figure B-1
Study Process

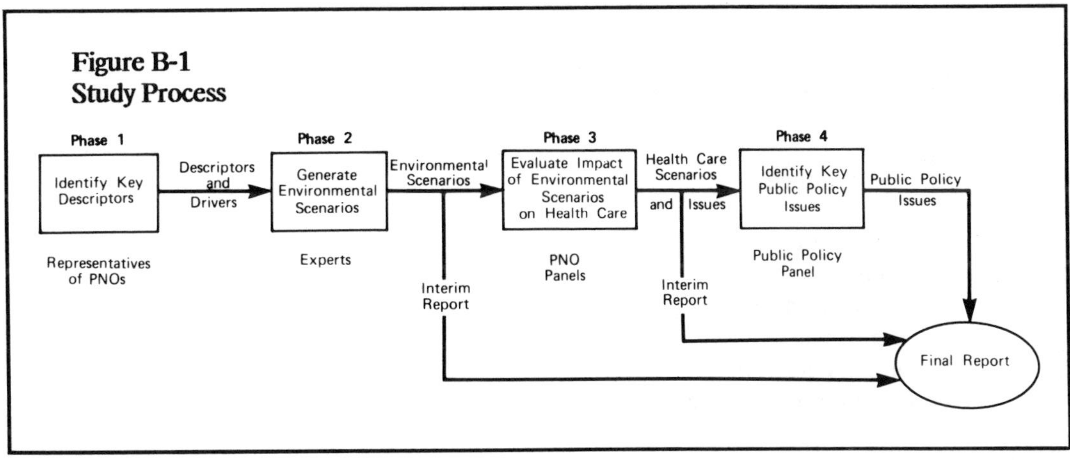

Figure B-2
Phase 1: Descriptors and Factors

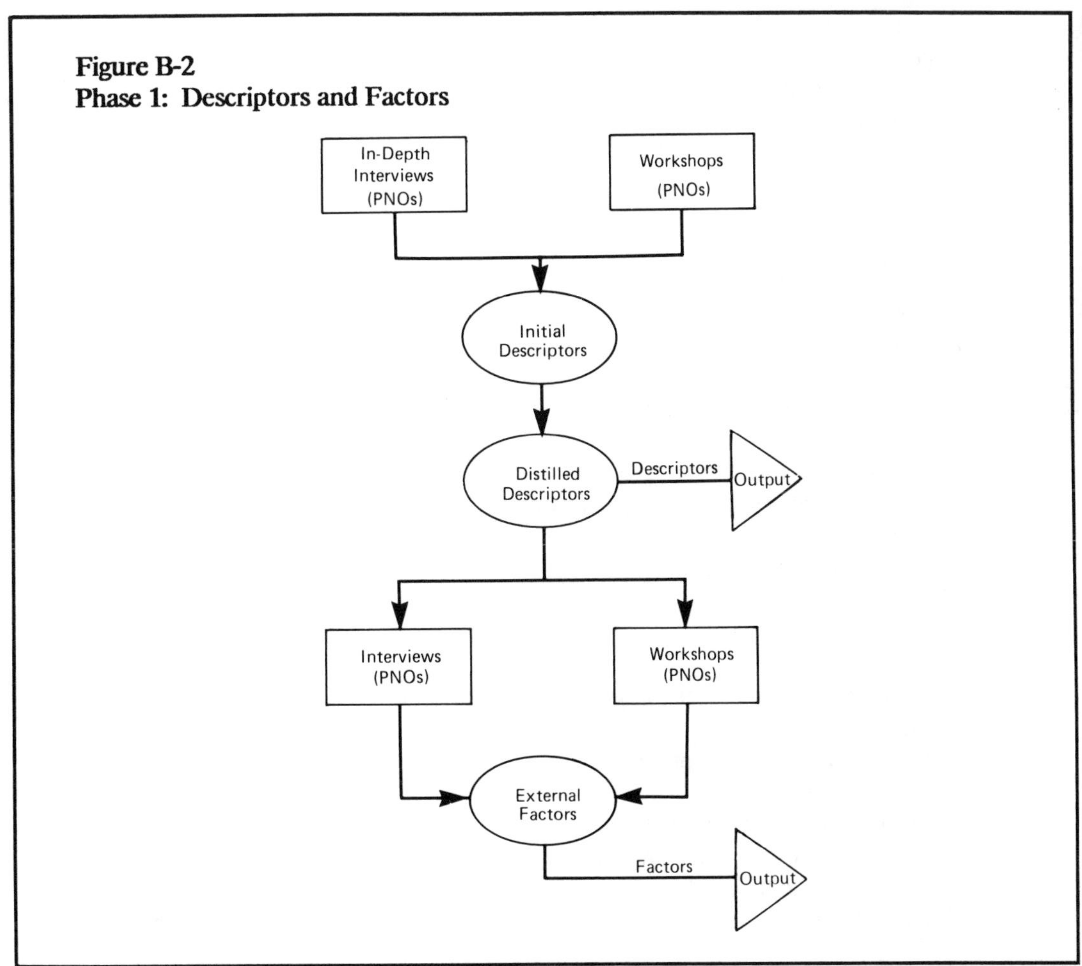

Table B-1
List of Key Environmental Factors

Economy
- Economic growth
- Inflation
- Real interest rates
- Investment
- Balance of trade
- Unemployment
- Union strength
- Employment in small business

Demography
- Total population
- Aged population
- Dependency ratio
- Urbanization
- Immigration

Households/Lifestyles
- Households
- Working women
- Working mothers
- Family stability
- Income distribution
- Percent of consumer expenditures on health care
- Poverty rate
- Family poverty rate
- Percent population without health care insurance
- Educational attainment
- Voluntary health hazards
- Diet index

Attitudes
- Support for social spending in government budgets
- Trust in government
- Attitude toward science and technology
- Attitude toward dying
- Attitude toward cost of health care
- Attitude toward medical providers
- Role of media in medical issues
- Entrepreneurship

..... continued

Table B-1
List of Key Environmental Factors (concluded)

Government
- Government spending
- Social spending by government: federal versus state/local
- Health program spending by government
- Percent health care spending by Medicare
- Environmental spending
- Budget deficit: federal versus state/local
- Volatility of government policy
- Regulation:
    - Control of doctors' clinical judgment
    - Interest rate subsidies for nonprofits
    - Financing of hospitals
    - Tax status of hospitals
    - Regulation of insurers
    - Prospects for NHI
    - Time lag between testing and payment by third-party payers
    - Use of technology for terminal patients

Technology
- R&D spending
- R&D spending by private sources
- Biotechnology sales
- Diffusion of doctor-intensive technologies
- Diffusion of take-home technologies
- Diffusion of information technology

Phase 2: Environmental Scenarios (Figure B-3)

The objective here was to develop the raw material from which our environmental forecasts could be generated. Using a set of individuals--selected because their expertise matched closely the set of environmental factors--we conducted one-on-one, face-to-face (two were done by telephone), in-depth interviews with each. The semistructured interviews were divided into three approximately equal part:

Part A. We asked the interviewees to scan our full list of factors/variables (see table B-1) and to identify about five or ten that they considered "crucial in shaping the future health care system." For most factors--if requested--we provided appropriate historical data.

Figure B-3
Phase 2: Environmental Scenarios

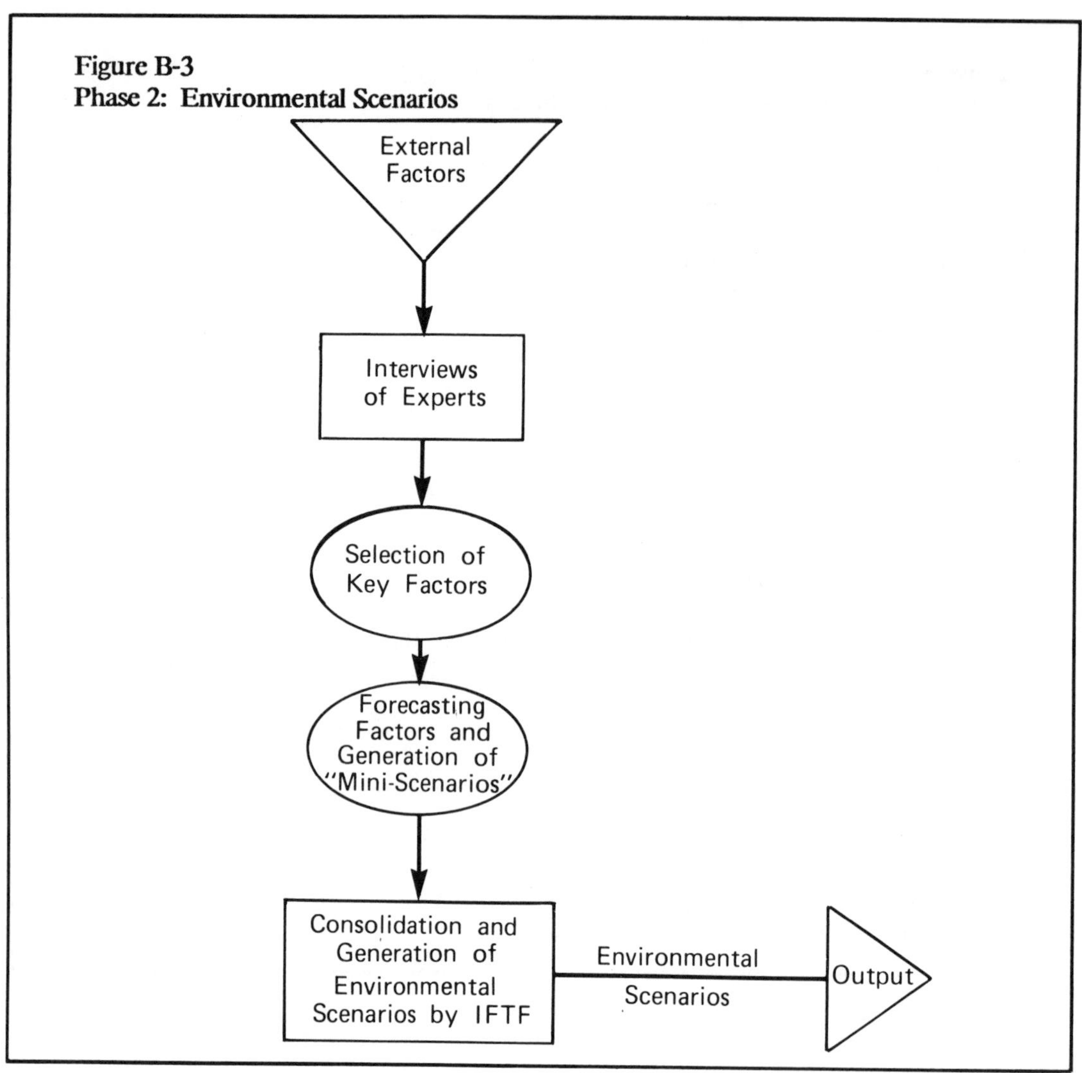

At least as important as the factors/variables selected by the interviewees were the detailed descriptions they provided of the rationale underlying their choices and the rationale underlying the perceived trends, factors, and interactions among forecasts (not all factors or variables were necessarily drawn from our list).

This process was repeated for each factor selected--in each case focusing on a "cluster" of interactions as described above. Each cluster represented a component of a larger scenario, a sort of mini-scenario, if you will.

Part B. The interviewees were asked to provide another set of descriptions for each of the factors selected in part A, this time conditional on a set of prescribed (that is, "what if") assumptions about the future health care system that we prepared. For example, one such assumption was: "Suppose the current efforts at cost containment are successful in keeping the fraction of GNP allocated to health care constant. Tell me what might have happened in the external environment that would be consistent with that outcome."

Another assumption provided was: "Suppose government, corporations, and insurers retreat from cost containment measures and that people are willing to pay whatever it costs for health care. Tell me how the outcome might occur." The result was not only the description of a "cluster" of interactions among external factors but also the connection to the prescribed outcome.

Part C. We asked the interviewees to make observations, raise questions, identify issues, and generally provide personal perceptions and views about likely changes, major uncertainties, possible surprises, and relatively implausible alternatives in the future health care environment.

This raw information--forecasts, clusters of interacting factors, and underlying "logical" connecting factors to prescribed health care outcomes--was used by IFTF to construct two plausible, internally consistent environmental scenarios that spanned the essential range of expert perceptions we had elicited.

SAMPLE RESPONSE No. 1

"This scenario is very likely. The reason for this view is that society adjusts well in the long run to problems it recognizes. The first generation corrections or trajectories now in place ultimately will be replaced by improvements that will be more successful. Further, older doctors are dying or retiring and younger doctors are now more awake and sensible about the issues. Also, most threats are near-term threats--with the danger that we may overreact. Once we get into the middle 1990s, we will see 'second generation' economic and political devices in place that capitalize on what is clearly the political will in this country--namely, to reduce health care expenditure growth."

SAMPLE REPONSE No. 2

"This scenario is plausible because, in spite of our efforts in the past fifteen years to contain health care costs, we have been unable to do so. Apparently, some powerful factors stand in the way and prevent us from reaching our objectives. Sure, hospital admission growth rates are down, but this was easy to achieve and was long overdue. However, the demand for ambulatory facilities is increasing. So, on net, health care expenditures will continue rising. This is a more realistic view of what is likely to take place. "Basically, the consumer likes the present health care system and wants more--and we have been educating the consumer to want more--in the form of long-term care coverage, ambulatory care, and preventive services. Also, technologically we can now do more. So we have both 'taste' and 'technological' imperatives operating. Government and industry efforts to curb health care expenditures will not be determining. The public will get what it wants. A leveling might not happen even if we face an economic disaster. Health is a domestic product produced by domestic resources that involves 8 million people. It might be viewed as a 'semirecession proof' industry."

Phase 3: Health Care Scenarios and Issues (Figure B-4)

The two environmental scenarios were used to provide the backdrop for extensions of these scenarios into the health care system. This was done as follows. Each PNO group was first provided the environmental scenarios for review. Each group was then assembled separately for a full-day workshop to:

- Modify and "flesh out" the scenarios where necessary.

- Make provisional forecasts of their relevant health care descriptors; for example, physician income for the physician group, hospital admissions for hospital administrators, and so forth) conditional on the assumptions of each scenario (historical data on all descriptors were provided).

- Adjust each forecast by interrelating individual forecasts.

- Describe the logic of each forecast.

The results of this first round were distilled, cross-checked, and integrated by IFTF into two consolidated health care scenarios (each an extension of the corresponding environmental scenario). These scenarios --with "cross-exchange" of information from PNO groups--were now provided again to each stakeholder group in a second set of full-day workshops to: review and "flesh out" each health care scenario; adjust each forecast and the logic of forecast interconnections; identify and rank issues--threats, opportunities, choices--that would need to be addressed as a result of changes in *either* or *both* scenarios.

The process of cross-checking is critical if scenarios are to be internally consistent. First, and most important, this process involves qualitative judgments by experts on whether forecasted variables would change in particular directions relative to one another. For example, experts would be asked to consider whether the forecasted number of hospital admissions was logically consistent with the basic demographic changes, number of insured, number of physicians, and so forth. Second, where possible, specific quantitative cross-checks are made using a number of mathematical identities that must hold in any scenario. For example, total government spending on health care (in dollar terms) must be mathematically consistent with the scenario-based assumptions of GNP, government share of GNP, and share of government expenditures allocated to the health care system. The principal task for the scenario writer is to fine-tune the forecast information using both logical and quantitative cross checks. To ensure the highest level of internal consistency, forecasts are reviewed on an iterative basis by expert groups--in this study by panels that were convened twice with each PNO group.

In the final step of Phase 3, we identified a set of health care issues. In some instances, these were evoked by each PNO group during discussions focused on a single scenario (for example, the substantial loss of physician autonomy in Scenario I). In other instances, issues were identified by examining and comparing effects "across" both scenarios (for example, increasing intensity of competition among hospitals). In still other instances, group members introduced topical issues de novo (for example, tax and antitrust changes affecting health insurers) and "played" them against each scenario. In each case, the scenarios served as internally consistent referents for examining and validating likely impacts on major actors.

The result of this phase was a final review of two health care scenarios and associated health care issues.

Figure B-4
Phase 3: Health Care Scenarios and Issues

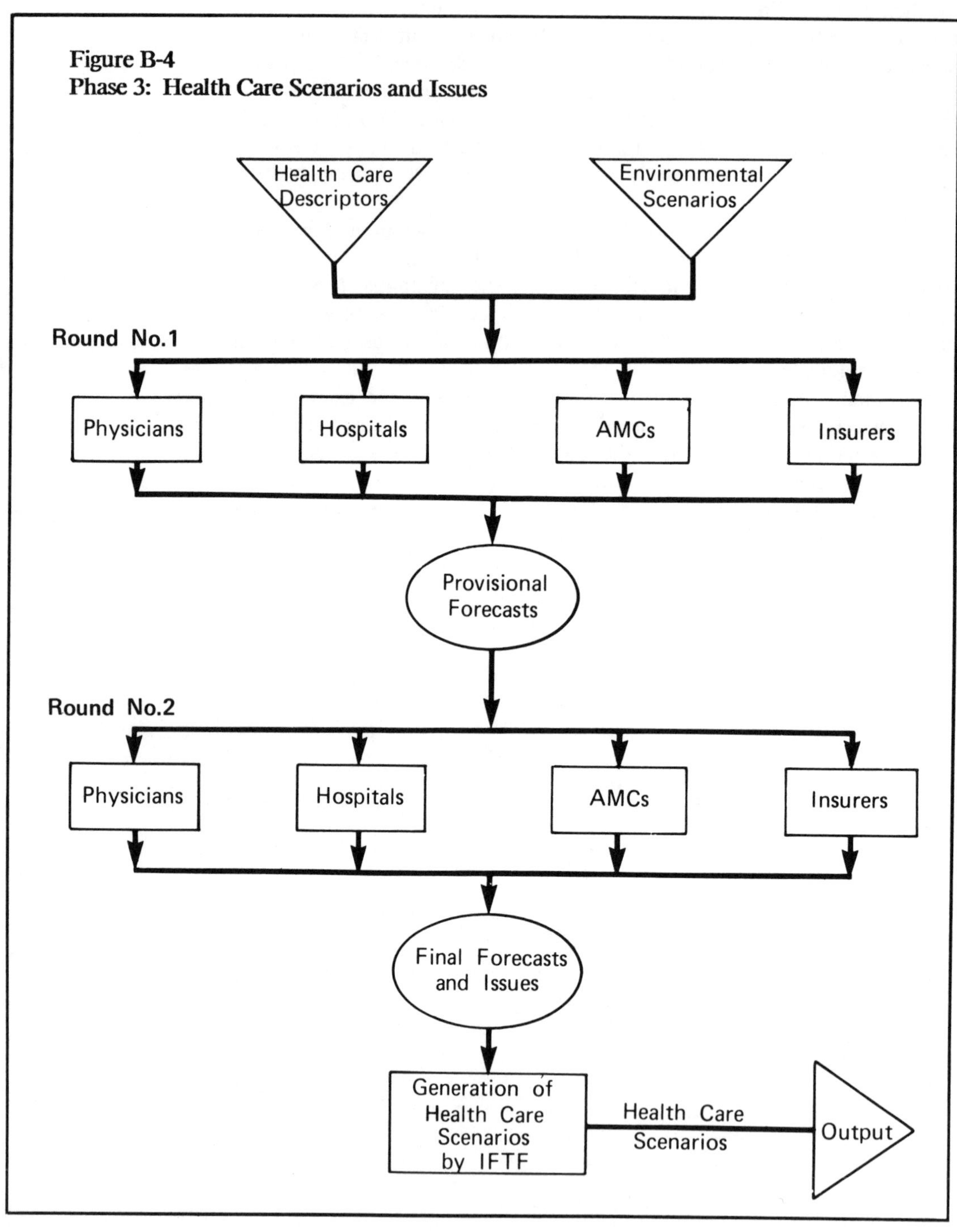

Phase 4: Public Policy Issues (Figure B-5)

The final phase of the study focused on forecasts of societal-level descriptors (for example, health status, cost, access, quality, government expenditures) and an overall review of study findings. In a full-day meeting of the Public Policy Panel, provisional forecasts of societal descriptors were adjusted and additions were made to the original list; overall study findings--environmental scenarios, health care scenarios and issues--were reviewed and critiqued (using the process described in Phase 3); and a set of public policy issues--related to but distinct from the health care issues generated by representatives of the PNOs--was identified.

Figure B-5
Phase 4: Public Policy Issues

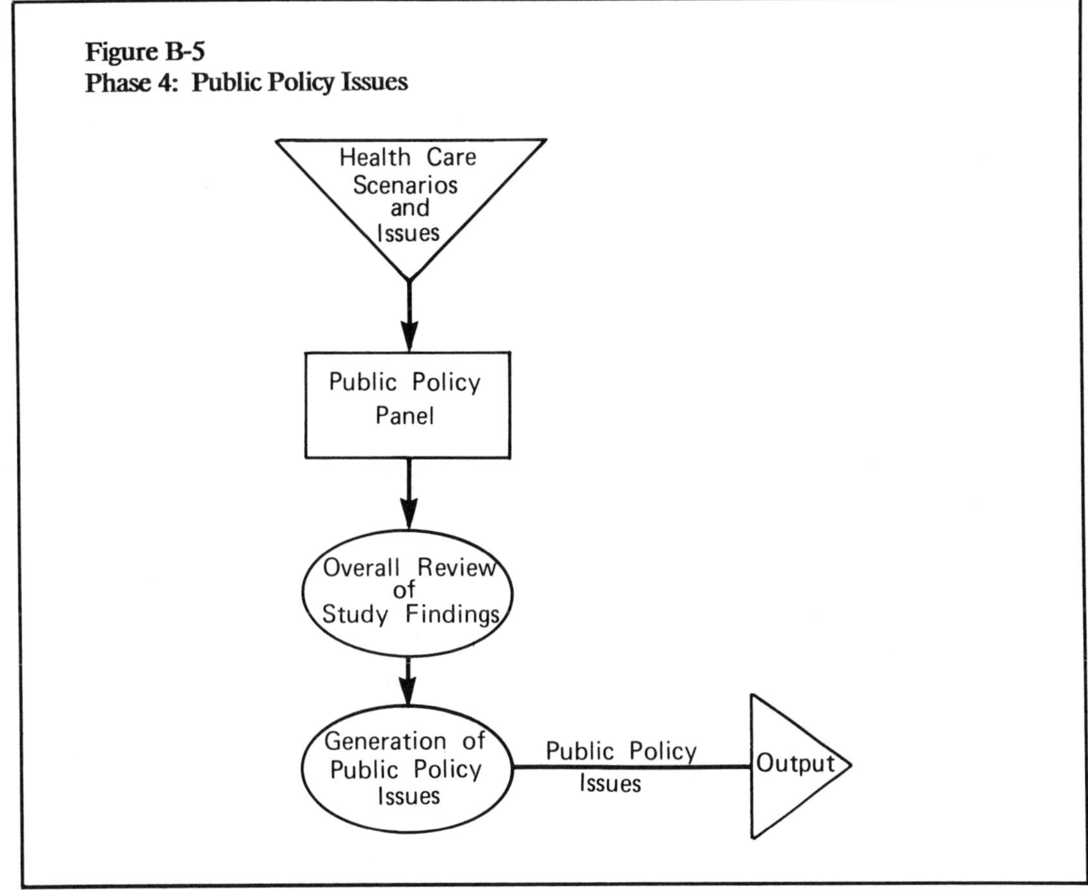

Appendix C

How to Use the Study

SCENARIO-BASED PLANNING AS A TOOL

Scenario-based planning with large numbers of participants is a unique and valuable tool in helping us prepare for an uncertain future. It is meant to deal with a basic human dichotomy: we can never know what the future will be and yet we must make decisions today on the basis of assumptions about that future. Scenario-based planning is a means of exploring opposing viewpoints about the future and using the insights gained to identify and set priorities for current decisions.

This book represents a process with four distinct steps. Each step is meant to present the reader with the considered viewpoints of experts and to engage the reader in examining his or her own assumptions in light of that group judgment. The goal of the effort, then, is not to convince the reader of a point of view but to help make key assumptions explicit and to help identify points of disagreement between the reader and the particular group of experts we have assembled. We hope this process of assumption checking will be a valuable contribution to the decision process which will shape the U.S. health care system of the 21st century.

There are four distinct steps in the process outlined in this book, and each step will engage the reader in redefining his or her assumptions.

1. Key driving forces. We used our experts to identify the forces that are most likely to cause change in the health care system over the next ten to fifteen years. They include those described in Chapter 1 and also include those embedded in our two scenarios, such as the aging of the baby boom cohort, attitudes toward government spending priorities, and profitability of business. This list of driving forces is not meant to be comprehensive, but rather it is intended to identify those forces that were considered most important by this particular group of experts.

2. Combinations of drivers. The key driving forces can be combined in any number of ways, with differing weights or relative importance attached to each. We generated two scenarios on the basis of a key outcome variable--the total amount of spending on health care. Each of the two chosen scenarios represents a plausible

outcome. The driving forces selected for each scenario are chosen to highlight the key differences between the scenarios. Thus, the factors that are common to both scenarios are not given as much weight as those that separate the scenarios. The scenarios are useful, then, not as forecasts of what will be, but as consistent pictures of what might result from the interplay of a particular set of driving forces. The reader may modify either of the scenarios as he or she sees fit.

3. Impacts on the health care system. Each scenario has a different impact on the health care system measured in terms of practice styles, hospital admissions, and the location of medical research. Again, the value of the impact scenarios is to present two consistent models linking driving forces and impacts on the system. The reader may modify any of the impact linkages and derive an independent set of linking assumptions to stimulate his or her thinking.

4. The key issues. The experts who had gone through the scenario exercise then identified the most important issues or choices which face the health care system. These issues are independent of a particular scenario, but reflect the insights of those who have gone through the process of building and discussing alternate scenarios. Again, the reader can test his or her own set of issues against those that result from this particular process.

Each of these four steps offers an opportunity for the reader to test his or her assumptions against those of a panel of experts.

EXAMPLES OF USES OF SCENARIOS

The goal of the book is not to describe what the future will look like but to engage readers in a process for examining one's assumptions about the future and for setting priorities on current choices. Three examples of utilizing scenarios for health care organizations are provided below. They illustrate different purposes at three different organizational levels.

Trustees, Boards, Top Management

The scenarios--in original or abbreviated form--can be effectively used by boards and senior organizational executives to help "rethink" basic organizational goals and missions. This may be done at annual "retreats" or "planning workshops" both through presentations and small group meetings in which active participation of attendees is encouraged. Both information and process are relevant here. The information contained in the scenarios can be used as points of departure for creating a "best guess" trajectory or for "extending" the scenarios to develop forecasts of descriptors of direct relevance to the organization. Also, the workshop processes described in Appendix B of this report can be replicated in small group sessions. One of the most useful "end products" from such exercises is the development of a shared vision to guide the organization's future development.

For example, the members of a hospital board strongly feel the need to develop a more coherent view of how the health care system is likely to change in the next ten to twenty years. In trying to set long-term directions for the hospital, it has become clear that the different members bring quite different "world views" of both the external environment shaping the health care system and the health care system itself. Some believe that the drop in hospital admissions is only a temporary phenomenon, while others feel it signals a major structural change; some feel the hospital must look outside traditional health care boundaries for income, while others feel it should stick "close to its knitting"; some feel that the resolve of business and government to contain costs will soon wane, while others do not. What is sought is an opportunity to construct an overall framework within which a common vision of the broad outlines of the health care system may evolve. The chairman suggests a one-day "mind-stretching" retreat for the twenty-member board. Here is a summary of what takes place.

Prior to the meeting, each member is provided a ten- to twenty-page summary of the two basic scenarios focusing exclusively on the environmental drivers (economy, demography, households and lifestyles, attitudes, role of government, and technology). Omitted is any information on how these contrasting external environments may change the health care system itself. In the first two hours of the retreat day, the environmental scenarios are described in detail to the full group. Ample opportunity is provided for questioning assumptions, the number of scenarios, the positioning of the scenarios, and possible "wild cards." The participants may reposition the scenarios, change basic assumptions, and fill in important gaps. The only restriction is that they aggregate their perceptions into two scenarios. This is the "buy-in" stage of the process.

Following the morning break, the group is assembled and challenged to construct their "best guess" single trajectory from the two elemental scenarios. If the scenarios resemble the two original ones presented, a great deal will turn on the degree of resolve of business and government in "enforcing" cost containment. In one such session, the consensus is that the current cost containment policies will eventually make themselves felt in the early 1990s but that the inexorable forces of aging and new technologies would eventually break the hold by the late 1990s. The resulting health care cost trajectory (that is, percent of GNP allocated to health care) falls between those of the two scenarios. Other trajectories are possible and also are discussed. The afternoon is devoted to assessing the impact of the chosen trajectory on the health care system and hospital activity.

Organization-wide or Association Planning Staffs

Most organizations of any size and virtually all industry, business, or professional associations have developed strong internal capabilities for forecasting and planning. For such organizations and groups, the study can be used to augment and extend internally available information and processes. This may be done in several ways:

- Extending planning horizons that often stop at the three-to-five-year horizon.

- Widening and deepening environmental forecasts that normally are "short-changed" in organizational planning processes.

- Developing a "map" of relevant issues so that interconnections among issues may be seen more clearly and priorities set more intelligently.

But perhaps the most important contribution that the study can make at this level is in helping to develop a clearer framework for connecting environmental and industry (or business) scenarios to the organization's option-generating and decisionmaking processes. A useful--and currently popular--vehicle for doing this is the "issue" construct. Analyses of issues can provide two kinds of information: (1) linkages back to the scenarios that identify high "value-added" information that needs to be collected or monitored; and (2) linkages forward to stimulate the generation of options or choices for confronting issues effectively.

For example, health care planners at federal, state, or county levels are generally quite familiar with the most important public policy issues confronting them. High on their list are issues of the so-called vulnerable populations dealing with the uninsured and underinsured, low-income women with children, long-term care for the elderly, and patients with AIDS. Public sector planners and administrators struggle with such issues day-to-day: they temporize, they fire fight, they improvise, and they hold their breath. What they generally lack--and desperately need--is an opportunity to view those issues from a more strategic standpoint; that is, the interrelationship of issues, their likely future trajectories, the trade-offs that may be made, and the priorities for addressing them.

The starting point here is a set of key issues. Either in small group settings or more formal workshops, the initial set can be expanded by using the two scenarios as backdrops for a more extended and integrated view of the health care system. The first result may be an "issue map" showing how the issues stem from particular environmental drivers and how they are related to each other. To this may now be added a "time line" (extending five to ten or more years) that shows how different issues develop over time. These are the first steps for estimating resource allocation (money, manpower, programs) requirements in aggregate form and for suggesting priorities. Using the scenarios, a number of "what if" questions are posed that are traced through the issue map. The result is the ability to see more coherently and explicitly the trade-offs to be evaluated when faced with limited resources, such as between low-income women with children and the elderly requiring long-term care (the so-called generational choices). Without the kind of "global view" that is provided by the scenarios and associated issues, such choices are obscure at best and unexamined at worst.

Line or Operating Managers

Hospital CEOs, divisional managers, or group heads are usually concerned with more regionalized or localized strategic issues--and associated options or choices--that confront them:

- How much should I spend on marketing?
- Should we joint venture with an HMO?
- What should I do with my excess beds?
- Is mental health an attractive opportunity for diversification?
- How can we develop "prevention and wellness" programs that will be attractive and profitable?

For such choices, the study can provide a valuable "reality check" and framework, provided appropriate linkages are constructed. The steps in this process include:

- Identifying the key external trends affecting each regional or local issue or choice.
- Determining whether regional or local trends are consistent with or different from national trends.
- Identifying the factors that account for the differences and similarities.
- Collecting historical data on regional or local trends and using these as a basis for making provisional forecasts that are extensions or variants of the original scenarios.
- Engaging line managers in workshops for evaluating issues and choices in the context of both local and national trends.

Using such processes, useful "bridges" can be built between national, macroenvironmental forecasts and the specific choices that line managers face.

For example, health care insurers, more so than other health care executives and managers, are caught in the middle between payers and providers. Almost all are struggling with a key choice: to what extent and how fast should we move toward managed care systems? Is managed fee-for-service the wave of the future, or are PPOs or HMOs destined to take the lion's share of the market? How can I hedge my strategy if we could be sure about the relative success of cost containment? Which regional markets should I concentrate on? What about timing?

In this instance, the path is from decision to be made back to the health care system and back to the basic environmental assumptions. In so doing, important gaps will almost surely have to be filled in. These may require acquiring relevant regional or local data on PPO and HMO growth to tie to national trends. Or the data may describe the latest trends on consumer or employee attitudes on managed care systems. The important point is that these backward linkages are added to a coherent framework of assumptions--any of which may be changed but whose effect by so doing may be explicitly examined.

In small group meetings or workshops, line managers and their staffs may be led through processes for examining the implications of such choices. The starting and ending point is the decision to be made. In between, the evaluation of the choice requires leading the group to underlying assumptions for each scenario about the structure of the health care system (for example, forecasts of managed fee-for-service, contract, and capitated care) and the external drivers shaping it. The key is that these assumptions "fit together" and are not the result of hit-or-miss selections of data or deliberate attempts to shape the outcome to suit preconceived perceptions. A possible choice that is suggested: a "hedged strategy" that opts for managed care through PPOs that may later evolve into capitated plans.

Appendix D

Important Medical Technologies: Selected Candidates for Change

Several interviews with experts focused exclusively on identifying technologies that are likely to have a major impact on medical care over the next ten to fifteen years. These technologies are listed in approximate order of their importance, as measured by the number of times experts mentioned them in their interviews:

1. Computers/Communications
2. Transplants/Artificial Organs/Prosthetics
3. Magnetic Resonance Imaging
4. Monoclonal Antibodies/DNA Probes
5. Endoscopy/In Vivo Monitoring
6. Home Diagnostic Tools
7. Drugs/Vaccines/Drug Delivery
8. Human Gene Therapy
9. Mental Health
10. Lasers
11. Surgical Advances
12. Positron Emission Tomography

Computers/communications. Improvements in this area include cheaper computer memory, miniaturization of the microprocessor and its peripherals, easier-to-use input/output functions such as voice recognition, and simplified networking among computers and electronic equipment. These advances will allow health care facilities to make wider use of computers in administration as well as patient care. Patient medical and financial records can be integrated into one database, for better resource planning and analysis. The record system can be hooked into an internal communications system, permitting remote access and updating from the nurse's station or from bedside, and even from automated patient monitoring equipment. Financial reporting among providers and payers can be automated and standardized. Three important aspects of medical computing will be:

- Decision Support Systems (DSS). Recent work has concentrated on developing expert system diagnostic aids (progress has been slow and spotty, but real gains are possible with simpler algorithms) and in administration and education. DSS's most important role may be to help payers monitor and exert control over choices of tests and procedures used in patient care.

However, the most exciting use of DSS will be in medical research. A well-designed DSS will link patient records on symptoms, treatments, and outcomes into a database that will let doctors discover the most cost-effective way to manage patients, not just a way to cut costs on current methods.

- Picture Archiving and Communication Systems (PACS). These systems translate diagnostic-related images into digital code, which permits image manipulation, electronic storage, and transmission. This capability could lower costs dramatically compared to storing film-based images, but initial equipment costs, lack of standardization, and, at present, the relatively poor quality of images have slowed PACS' diffusion. However, these systems are likely to have a major impact in the 1990s, particularly when used in conjunction with computerized decision systems, when they can reduce the need for test duplication, compare images from different types of equipment, and allow computer analysis of images.

- Computer-Aided Design (CAD). Computers can be used to model hypothetical systems before they are actually created, permitting testing and experimentation on paper (or on disk) before expensive prototypes are built. Designers are already using this technology to test drug molecules against receptors in the body, and in the design of individually tailored prosthetics. Computer-aided design can be extended to implanted organs and sensory aids, surgical simulations, and genetic manipulation.

Transplants/artificial organs/prosthetics. Transplants and transplant patient survival will increase greatly as we gain better understanding of immune system functions. Immunosuppressive drugs and procedures (cyclosporine, whole body irradiation) will increase acceptance of foreign tissue, and improvements in human tissue cloning (already begun with skin and retinal tissue) will allow patients to receive compatible transplants. Some of the most exciting work is in brain tissue transplants, using fetal or adrenal brain cells to augment functions impaired by such diseases as Parkinson's and Alzheimer's. At the same time, better artificial organs and prosthetics are being developed. Stronger, lightweight, biocompatible materials such as collagen and "bioglass" can be used in place of bone and cartilage, and manipulated by neural control through electrical stimulation. Sensory aids for vision and hearing will be miniaturized enough to be implanted as artificial eyes and ears.

Magnetic resonance imaging (MRI). MRI is the use of radio waves and strong magnetic fields to detect physical and chemical variations among tissues. It is used primarily for studies of the head and the nervous and cardiovascular systems. However, because of its safety advantages (no ionizing radiation) and ongoing rapid technical breakthroughs, MRI has a broad range of potential uses that compete with X rays, contrast imaging, CT scans, and spectroscopy. Several problems remain. Among them are the current high cost of operation, both in original equipment costs and in the skilled labor time needed to process a patient, and the inexperience of doctors at using and interpreting the images. However, the ability to image chemical changes as well as physical ones makes it the most exciting imaging technology, and functional improvements in size and image speed are already occurring.

Monoclonal antibodies (MAb)/DNA probes. Monoclonal antibody technology involves the fusing of a cancer cell with another cell that produces an antibody. The resulting "hybridoma" combines a cancer cell's propagation with the second cell's ability to produce useful antibodies. While the technology is still young, in theory MAbs can be developed for almost anything that evokes an antibody response, not just infectious diseases. Thus, they can be used to monitor drug levels in the body for diabetics or chemotherapy patients, detect the presence and levels of hormones for birth control and fertility assistance, or deliver substances to targeted body sites so that they show up better in X rays or receive concentrated doses of drugs. Factors needed for rapid growth of this technology include scaling up production and regulatory approval of the application of this technology in-vivo.

In contrast to MAbs, DNA probes are used strictly with genetic material. The identity of a given sample can be determined if a DNA strand of a known sequence hybridizes with DNA in the sample being tested. Such probes can be used to identify infectious diseases, the presence of drugs, prenatal abnormalities, and even disease susceptibility. DNA probes have the potential to displace many existing tests and to develop more information about certain disease states. However, there are still large gaps in theory linking specific diseases to the DNA that is being measured and, as with MAbs, production is still expensive and difficult.

Endoscopy/in-vivo monitoring. This technology uses a small catheter in a blood vessel or body cavity to perform an examination or test, to extract a specimen, or to deliver a contrast medium to an imaging site. The catheter can convey a laser for surgery or a microprocessor to evaluate conditions or even to guide the endoscope. Current developments include expansions in sensor technology, continuous in-vivo spectroscopy, and closed-loop systems that can detect and correct various conditions.

Some diagnostic uses of endoscopy are being replaced by techniques that are still less invasive. For example, arteriography (use of catheters to deliver contrast media to a blood vessel for an enhanced X ray image) is being replaced by noninvasive, computer-enhanced contrast imaging systems, which themselves ultimately will be replaced by MRI. However, endoscopy will remain an important technology for at least the next ten years.

Home diagnostic tools. This category includes all tools and kits that are sold over the counter to households for diagnostic use. Such products can be used to monitor the status of chronic conditions such as diabetes or to act as a screening device to decide whether a doctor's visit is appropriate. The home market is potentially huge, and at least some of the tests would add to, rather than substitute for, tests provided today. The growth in use will be limited by several factors: questions about the reliability of the tests, the expertise needed to use them properly, and increased out-of-pocket costs (since home tests are not included within the current reimbursement schemes).

Home testing will benefit from developments in immunochemical testing and improvements in reliability that are affecting all diagnostics. For example, monoclonal antibody tests shorten the time for tests, standardize the results, and make them easier to interpret. Use of dry-chemistry, film-based tests will spread from labs and doctors' offices to homes as the level of skill needed to perform the tests drops and automated film readers move into pharmacies. Dipsticks that change color on detecting chemicals in blood or urine will allow many tests to be done immediately, allowing treatment to begin without waiting for results from the lab.

Drugs/vaccines/drug delivery. There are four generators of change in the drug area: (1) basic biochemical research, (2) computers, (3) biotechnology, and (4) drug delivery systems. Improvements in the biochemical understanding of body metabolism and function mean that drugs can be more precisely tailored to the body's needs. Computerized design makes it possible to tailor drugs quickly, modeling and testing many compounds before selecting those likely to be most effective. Computer-based expert systems can assist with drug therapy, particularly for compounds with very narrow ranges for safe use. Biotechnology advances create new processes for drug production, particularly for vaccines via the creation of extremely specific monoclonal antibodies. Finally, improvements in drug delivery include controlled release to prevent peaks and valleys in drug levels in the body, targeted delivery via monoclonal antibodies or liposome carriers, implantable pumps, and improvements in transdermal applications.

Human gene therapy. Rather than providing drugs from outside the body, human gene therapy would alter the functioning of the body itself by inserting, removing, or modifying the person's own genetic material. Only new gene insertion is likely in the short run and will involve adding genes to change enzyme production. Likely first applications will be in metabolic diseases, sickle cell anemia, and the thalassemias.

Mental health. Recent research has indicated that many of the more serious disorders such as schizophrenia are biochemically based. Basic research in the neurochemistry of brain function (including the use of positron emission tomography scans, see below) will provide understandings of the processes that go awry and the appropriate drugs or gene therapy to correct them. For less serious mental disease, improvements in counseling will come from better training, including the use of computer simulations such as "Parry" (a "paranoid" program).

Lasers. Lasers are tightly focused, high-power light sources that are converted to heat at their target point. They can be routed along optical fibers in endoscopes for diagnosis and surgery within the body or used outside for drug activation or surgery. (Similar capabilities are being developed with microwaves.)

Surgical advances. New techniques and instrumentation will reduce the trauma from surgery and speed healing. Using lasers or miniature instruments threaded through endoscopes reduces the size of the opening into the body and reduces blood loss and the risk of infection. Such techniques also make in-utero surgery on the fetus possible. Lasers and microwave scalpels will minimize blood loss. In-vivo sensors and real-time imaging permit constant monitoring of the patient's status during the operation, and better wound-closing materials (such as improved sutures and biocompatible glues) will permit faster healing.

Positron emission tomography (PET). This technology is an imaging tool that tracks the gamma rays produced from positron-electron annihilation of a positron-emitting compound injected into the body. PET images biochemical processes rather than physical structure and so has excellent research potential for understanding brain and other organ functions. However, its high cost and unwieldy process may limit any wider use. Rather, PET will establish metabolic understanding, allowing simpler MRI-based tests to be developed. An important offshoot is SPECT (Single Photon Emission CT), which does not require a cyclotron for positron creation and can be used as a simple imaging system.

Appendix E

Table E-1
Wild Cards

Description	Experts Mentioned	PNO Participants Mentioned
Technology		
1. A major breakthrough in the treatment of cancer.	2	3
2. An ability to dissolve clots in coronary artery disease.		1
3. A major breakthrough in cost-effective preventive medicine.	1	
4. The development of new drugs with an impact like penicillin.	1	
5. A dramatic jump in longevity of humans.	1	
6. The ability of humans to "grow their own" heart.	1	
7. Control of the aging process.	1	
8. A breakthrough in treatment using monoclonal antibodies.	1	
9. Spin-offs from the Strategic Defense Initiative/impact on innovation.	1	
10. Breakthroughs in genetic engineering.	1	
11. Little or no progress in research.		1
12. Success in xenogeneic organ transplants.		1
Organization		
13. Malpractice crisis escalates.	1	
14. Physicians form a doctors' union.	1	
15. A dramatic change occurs in medical education, either length or type.	1	
16. Many academic medical centers fall into deep trouble.	1	
17. A low-cost, decentralized, technology-based system of health care delivery is successfully developed.	1	

. . . .continued

Table E-1
Wild Cards (concluded)

Description	Experts Mentioned	PNO Participants Mentioned
18. Health care delivery is conducted solely in the ambulatory setting.	1	
19. Allied health professions become major providers.		1
20. Physician unemployment becomes significant.		1
21. The Blues get heavily into life insurance.	1	
Epidemiology		
22. AIDS or AIDS-like diseases proliferate.	3	2
23. Mental health (demands and technology) explodes.	1	
24. The use of tobacco, drugs, and alcohol is eliminated.		1
Role of Government		
25. National health insurance is enacted.	3	4
26. The VA health care system is scrapped.	1	
27. COBRA-like legislation for the uninsured is dramatically extended.	1	
28. Hospitals lose their tax-exempt status.		1
29. Government introduces explicit rationing by age and income.		1
30. Federal and state governments split out health and welfare, each taking one.		1
31. Major shortfall occurs in Social Security trust funds.		1
32. Price controls are placed on the total health care system.		1
Other External Events		
33. Major nuclear accident stretches health care system and highlights inadequacies of disaster plans.		1
34. Sustained economic depression occurs.		1
35. War in Central America diverts funds from health.		1
36. All banks default.		1

Appendix F

Summary Tables

COMPARATIVE SUMMARY OF SCENARIOS

Table F-1
External Environment

Indicator	1985	2000 I	2000 II
Real GNP (average annual growth rate for preceding 15 years)	2.6	2.5	3.0
Real GNP (trillions of 1985 dollars)	4.00	5.80	6.23
Government spending (percent of GNP)	35.1	36.0	38.0
Attitudes toward diffusion of medical technologies	Expansive	Targeted Technologies	Expansive
Business health care expenditures as percent of total compensation	4.4	5.1	5.9
Percent GNP to health care	10.7	10.7	12.7

Table F-2
Health Care System

Indicator	1985	2000 I	2000 II
Total health care spending (billions of 1985 dollars)	425	622	790
Sources of health care expenditures (percent):			
Government	41.2	42.8	42.0
Business	29.0	28.1	28.4
Consumers	27.2	28.1	27.2
Private (other)	2.7	1.0	2.4
Health care structure (percent):			
Out of system	10	9	4
Fee-for-service	72	40	63
Contract	8	23	17
Capitated	10	28	16
Physician services per capita (1985 dollars)	390	407	546
Mean fee per physician visit (1985 dollars)	28	28	33.3
Hospital costs (percent of average weekly earnings)	153.9	160.0	185.0
Share of health expenditures to program Administration and net cost of insurance (percent)	6.2	7.0	6.2
Penetration of technology (percent of U.S. community hospitals):			
CT scanners	56	70	79
Cardiac catheterization	18	30	36
Organ transplant	5	9	17
Medical care variation (highest/lowest in 13 sites):			
Coronary artery bypass	3.1 (1981)	1.3	2.5
Total hip replacement	3.0 (1981)	1.4	2.5
Diagnostic upper GI	1.6 (1981)	1.2	1.5

.....continued

Table F-2
Health Care System (concluded)

Indicator	1985	2000 I	2000 II
Consumer satisfaction with health care (percent very/somewhat satisfied)	72	70	70
Infant mortality rates	10.8 (1984)	7.9	7.9
Prevention index*	63.2	69	72
Health care employment (millions)	6.3	9.1	10.7

*An index ranging from 0 indicating that no one had taken any preventive steps to 100 where everyone interviewed had taken all reasonable preventive steps in 21 specific health promotion behaviors.

Table F-3
Physicians

Indicator	1985	2000 I	2000 II
Number of active physicians (including Federal)	511,090	637,000	650,000
Number of new physicians per year	21,000	17,600	21,000
Average physician income in 1985 dollars (excluding residents)	113,000	96,000	118,000
Percent physicians on salary (including residents)	32.9	50.6	37.9
Share of health care spending:			
Billions of 1985 dollars	93.1	105.4	162.4
Percent	21.9	16.9	20.6
Distribution of income and expenses (billions of 1985 dollars):			
Physician income	48.8	54.7	74.8
Physician expenses	34.8	35.2	70.9
Lab costs/other costs	9.5	15.5	16.7

Table F-4
Hospitals

Indicator	1985	2000 I	2000 II
Total admissions (millions)	33.5	30.7	36.5
Admissions per 1,000 (number)	141	115	136
Length of stay (number of days)	7.1	7.0	7.1
Patient days (millions)	238	215	259
Patient days per 1,000 (number)	1,004	805	966
Number of beds (thousands)	1,003	818	1,009
Occupancy rate (percent)	65	72	70
Beds in small hospitals (percent of total)	14.2	8.0	11.0
Inpatient/outpatient revenue split (percent)	84/16	69/31	74/26
Uncompensated care (percent of revenues)	6	6	3
Total hospital services (billions of 1985 dollars)	156.4	245.1	288.0
Hospital share of total health care spending (percent)	36.8	39.3	36.5
Inpatient expenditure per acute care admission (1985 dollars)	3,343	4,847	5,049
Hospital costs (as percentage of average weekly earnings)	153.9	160	185

Table F-5
Academic Medical Centers

Indicator	1985	2000 I	2000 II
Number of U.S. medical schools	127	120	127
Number of medical school applicants (thousands)	32.9	27.0	31.3
Applicants per 1,000 target population	1.6	1.6	1.9
Accepted applicants (thousands)	17.2	15.7	17.2
Applicant/acceptance ratio	1.9	1.7	1.8
Newly licensed MDs (thousands)	21.0	17.6	21.0
Percent FMGs of newly licensed MDs	23.1	16.5	20.0
Medical school income (billions of 1985 dollars)	11.0	13.3	17.4
Percent of medical school income from own revenues	41	44	44
Percent of all patient activities in teaching hospitals:			
Inpatient days	21.4	22.4	23.3
Outpatient visits	30.0	28.9	29.4
Research spending (billions of 1985 dollars)	0.19	0.18	0.20
Research concentration (percent research in top 20 medical schools)	50	56	56

Table F-6
Insurers

Indicator	1985	2000 I	2000 II
Market share of top four commercial insurers (percent)	19	23	23
Market share of traditional insurers in managed care:			
Contract (percent)	76	75	75
Capitated (percent)	30	56	60
Uninsured population (millions)	35	32	16
Uninsured population (percent)	15	12	6
Program administration and net cost of insurance (billions of 1985 dollars)	26.2	45.0	49.0
Government health spending (billions of 1985 dollars):	174.8	267.0	332.0
Medicare	72.3	116.0	140.2
Medicaid	41.8	63.0	71.2
Other (including R&D, construction, and public health)	60.7	88.0	120.6

Appendix G

Glossary

Capitated: A method of reimbursement in which a provider receives a fixed fee per person from a defined population for a period of time, regardless of the number of services used by the enrollee.

Cafeteria Plans: Analogous to flexible benefits plans but where employees have a wide range of choice over which benefits are covered and the levels of coverage of those benefits.

COBRA: The Consolidated Omnibus Budget Reconciliation Act of 1986 requires employers who maintain health care plans to permit former employees, divorced and widowed spouses of employees, and former dependent children of employees to continue health care coverage at group rates for specified periods of time.

Contract: Arrangements in which providers deliver a group of services for a set fee or deliver individual services at negotiated discounts. Included are PPO arrangements and DRG-type reimbursement systems.

DRG: Diagnostic Related Group, a hospital patient classification system currently used to pay for Medicare patients. The federal government sets a predetermined price for a "package of hospital care" for each DRG.

Environmental Factor: A characteristic of the external environment over which little or no control can be exercised by the health care system but that may have considerable influence in shaping that system; e.g., economic growth rates, government spending, attitude toward dying.

FFS: Fee-for-service, a method of reimbursement in which physicians and hospitals are paid a "reasonable or customary fee" for a unit of service. Included are comprehensive first-dollar coverage, arrangements with deductibles and copayments, or plans using utilization reviews and mandatory second opinions.

Flexible Benefits Plan: A flexible benefits plan offers employees certain choices between different benefits packages, the right to include or exclude specific benefits such as a dental plan, or the right to trade health care benefits for other kinds of benefits.

Half-way Technology: Technology that "can compensate for the incapacitating effects of certain diseases" but cannot cure. Examples include transplantation of hearts, kidneys, livers, lungs, and implantation of artificial organs as well as kidney dialysis and bypass surgery. Such technologies are often very expensive and very much in demand.

Health Care Descriptor: A characteristic of the health care system that provides information about the "state" of the system. Examples are hospital admissions, number of uninsured, and average physician income.

HMO: Health Maintenance Organization, a health care providing organization that may have a closed group of physicians along with either its own hospitals or allocated beds in one or more hospitals. Patients are provided medical and hospital care on a capitated basis.

IPA: Independent Physician Association, a provider organization of physicians in which they maintain their own practices but agree to furnish services to patients who have signed up for a prepayment plan, such as in a capitated system.

Issue: A problem or concern (sometimes expressed as a threat or opportunity) created by a development or confluence of developments. Issues generally imply the need for identifying and evaluating appropriate choices to be made.

Managed Care: A broad spectrum of health delivery arrangements from fee-for-service with employer or insurer review through a full-service, integrated, "bricks and mortar" HMO.

PNO: Any of four Participating National Organizations in this study--American Medical Association, American Hospital Association, Association of American Medical Colleges, and Blue Cross/Blue Shield Association.

PPO: Preferred provider option, a form of insurance in which certain physicians and hospitals are identified by a third-party payer as preferred providers. These providers offer discounts in return for an expectation of increased volume. Beneficiaries receiving care from such physicians or hospitals incur lower out-of-pocket costs than traditional fee-for-service plans.

Scenario: An internally consistent description of a plausible future.

Triple Option: Hybrid health insurance options offered by employers that include an HMO, a PPO, and traditional indemnity insurance with utilization reviews.

Appendix H

Sources for Figures and Tables

FIGURES

Figure 1: U.S. Health Care Spending
Historical data: *Health Care Financing Review,* Fall 1985, p.3.

Figure 2: Changing U.S. Age Distribution
"Projections of the Population of the United States, by Age, Sex, and Race: 1983 to 2080," Series P-25, No. 952, Middle Series, U.S. Department of Commerce, Bureau of the Census.

Figure 3: Educational Attainment: Percent Population with 4+ Years of College
Historical data: Bureau of the Census, Current Population Reports, "Educational Attainment in the United States," Series P-20, various years.

Figure 4: Households with Children Under 18
Historical data: "Household and Family Characteristics," Series P-20, U.S. Department of Commerce, Bureau of the Census, various years.

Figure 5: Real GNP Growth
Historical data: U.S. Department of Commerce, Bureau of Economic Analysis, "U.S. National Accounts."

Figure 6: Government Deficit
Historical data: U.S. Department of Commerce, Bureau of Economic Analysis, "U.S. National Accounts."

Figure 7: Government Share of GNP
Historical data: U.S. Department of Commerce, Bureau of Economic Analysis, "U.S. National Accounts."

Figure 8: Public Confidence in Leaders of Institutions
Historical data: Compendium of Harris and NORC polls, various years, *Public Opinion,* April-May 1985.

Figure 9: Public Spending: Public Priorities
NORC General Social Surveys, 1984-1986 Combined, *Public Opinion,* May-June 1987.

Figure 10: Burden of Health Care Costs on Business
Historical data: U.S. Department of Commerce, Bureau of Economic Analysis, "U.S. National Accounts."

Figure 11: The Flow of Payments in the Health Care System
IFTF.

Figure 12: U.S. Health Care Spending
See Figure 1.

Figure 13: Public Confidence in Science
Historical data: National Science Foundation Annual Report, citing various published surveys.

Figure 14: The Growing Number of Elderly
See Figure 2.

Figure 15: Education Gap Narrows
Historical data and projection: Special Studies Series P-23, #13B, "Demographic and socioeconomic aspects of aging in the United States," U.S. Department of Commerce, Bureau of the Census, p. 99.

Figure 16: Working Women: Baby-Boom Households Have No Time to Care for Elderly Parents
Historical data and projections to 1995: "Employment Projections for 1995," U.S. Department of Labor, Bureau of Labor Statistics, Bulletin 2197, March 1984. (Forecasts based on high-growth projections for 1995.)

Figure 17: Government Share of GNP
Historical data: U.S. Department of Commerce, Bureau of Economic Analysis, "U.S. National Accounts."

Figure 18: Real GNP Growth, 1950-2000
See Figure 5.

Figure 19: Burden of Health Care Costs on Business
Historical data: U.S. Department of Commerce, Bureau of Economic Analysis, "U.S. National Accounts."

Figure 20: Physicians on Salary
Historical data: American Medical Association.

Figure 21: Physicians on Salary
See Figure 20.

Figure 22: Hospital Admissions
Historical data: American Hospital Association, *Hospital Statistics,* 1986 edition, page 3 for total nonfederal, short-term general, and other special hospitals.

Figure 23: Outpatient Revenues
Historical data: American Hospital Association, *Hospital Statistics,* various years.

Figure 24: Hospital Admissions
See Figure 22.

Figure 25: Outpatient Revenues
See Figure 23.

Figure 26: Newly Licensed Physicians
Historical data: *Statistical Abstract of the United States.*

Figure 27: Research Concentration
Historical data: estimates from panel participants.

Figure 28: Newly Licensed Physicians
See Figure 26.

Figure 29: Research Concentration
See Figure 27.

Figure 30: Penetration of Technology
Historical data: American Hospital Association, *Hospital Statistics,* 1981, 1986.

Figure 31: Consumer Satisfaction with Quality Health Care
Historical data: Louis Harris and Associates, *A Report Card on HMOs,* prepared for the Henry J. Kaiser Foundation.

Figure 32: Penetration of Technology
See Figure 30.

Figure 33: Consumer Satisfaction with Quality Health Care
See Figure 31.

APPENDIX FIGURES

Figure B-1: Study Process
IFTF.

Figure B-2: Phase 1: Descriptors and Factors
IFTF.

Figure B-3: Phase 2: Environmental Scenarios
IFTF.

Figure B-4: Phase 3: Health Care Scenarios and Issues
IFTF.

Figure B-5: Phase 4: Public Policy Issues
IFTF.

TABLES

Table 1: Government Tax Receipts
Historical data: U.S. Department of Commerce, Bureau of Economic Analysis, "U.S. National Accounts."

Table 2: Retained Business Profits
Historical data: U.S. Department of Commerce, Bureau of Economic Analysis, "U.S. National Accounts."

Table 3: People Favoring the Right to Die for Those with Incurable Diseases
Public Opinion, August/September 1985.

Table 4: Government Spending
Historical data: U.S. Department of Commerce, Bureau of Economic Analysis, "U.S. National Accounts."

Table 5: National Health Expenditures: Source of Funds
Historical data: National Health Accounts, *Health Care Financing Review*.

Table 6: The Changing Structure of U.S. Health Care
Historical data: "Out of System" based on estimates derived from various sources reported in *The Washington Post,* National Weekly Edition, July 21, 1986, p. 9; in *Hospitals,* October 20, 1986, pp. 46-51; and in *The New York Times,* January 13, 1986, p. 1. "Fee for Service" based on estimates derived from National Accounts of Health Expenditures, *Health Care Financing Review,* Fall 1986; and from Wyatt Company Survey of Corporate

Health Benefits, cited in *Medical Benefits,* November 15, 1986. "Contract Care" estimated from data cited in 1986 Survey of Multiunit Providers, *Modern Health Care,* June 1986, and *California Hospital Fact Book,* 1986, for PPO Membership and National Accounts Data (see above) for DRG coverage. "Capitated" was derived from Interstudy's Report on HMOs, July 1986.

Table 7: Relative Shares of Health Care Spending
Historical data: *Health Care Financing Review,* Fall 1986 (HCFA); American Medical Association, *Socioeconomic Characteristics of Medical Practice,* 1985. (Characteristics, AMA.)

Table 8: Voters in Presidential Elections by Age
Historical data: "Voting and Registration," *Current Population Reports,* Population Characteristics Series P-20, U.S. Department of Commerce, Bureau of the Census, various years. Recent age specific voting patterns were applied to middle series population projections to generate forecasts.

Table 9: Top Ten Swing States in Presidential Elections
Historical data and population projections: see Figure 2. Electoral College data from *Statistical Abstract of the United States.*

Table 10: Government Spending
Historical data: U.S. Department of Commerce, Bureau of Economic Analysis, "U.S. National Accounts."

Table 11: Government Spending
Historical data: U.S. Department of Commerce, Bureau of Economic Analysis, "U.S. National Accounts."

Table 12: The Tax Burden
Bureau of Economic Analysis.

Table 13: Government Tax Receipts
Historical data: U.S. Department of Commerce, Bureau of Economic Analysis, "U.S. National Accounts."

Table 14: National Health Expenditures: Source of Funds
Historical data: National Health Accounts, *Health Care Financing Review.*

Table 15: Government Spending (All Levels)
See Table 10.

Table 16: Health Care Expenditures: Sources of Funds
National Health Accounts, *Health Care Financing Review*.

Table 17: Consumer Expenditures on Health Care
Statistical Abstract of the United States, 1987, Table 135, citing U.S. Bureau of Labor Statistics, Consumer Expenditure Survey: Interview Survey.

Table 18: Total Health Care Spending: National Health Accounts
Historical data: See Table 7.

Table 19: Structure of U.S. Health Care
Historical data: See Table 6.

Table 20: Service Expansion
IFTF.

Table 21: Number of Active Physicians
Historical data: *Statistical Abstract of the United States;* Characteristics, AMA.

Table 22: Number of Physicians by Major Type of Activity
Historical data: *Statistical Abstracts* and *California Hospital Fact Book.*

Table 23: Physician Specialties
Historical data: Characteristics, AMA.

Table 24: Physician Income
Historical data: Characteristics, AMA; National Health Accounts, HCFA.

Table 25: Number of Active Physicians
See Table 21.

Table 26: Physician Income
See Table 24.

Table 27: Number of Physicians by Major Type of Activity
See Table 22.

Table 28: Physicians: Comparative Summary of Scenarios
As previously referenced.

Table 29: Hospital Activity Descriptors
Historical data: American Hospital Association, *Hospital Statistics.*

Table 30: Hospital Beds and Occupancy Rates
Historical data: American Hospital Association, *Hospital Statistics.*

Table 31: Beds in Small Hospitals
Historical data: American Hospital Association, *Hospital Statistics.*

Table 32: Hospitals' Distribution of Total Health Care Spending
Historical data: National Health Accounts, *Health Care Financing Review,* Fall 1986; and *Hospital Statistics,* American Hospital Association, 1986.

Table 33: Hospital Activity Descriptors
See Table 29.

Table 34: The Aging of the Elderly
See Figure 2.

Table 35: Hospital Beds and Occupancy Rates
See Table 30.

Table 36: Beds in Small Hospitals
See Table 31.

Table 37: Hospitals' Distribution of Total Health Care Spending
See Table 32.

Table 38: Hospitals: Comparative Summary of Scenarios
As previously referenced.

Table 39: Number of Fully Accredited and Provisionally Accredited U.S. Medical Schools
Historical Data: *Data Book,* Association of American Medical Colleges, Series A1.

Table 40: Applicants and Acceptances to Medical Schools
Historical data: *Data Book,* Association of American Medical Colleges, Series B 1. Population data and projections: U.S. Bureau of the Census.

Table 41: Medical School Income
Historical data: *Data Book,* Association of American Medical Colleges, Series D1.C.

Table 42: Sources of Medical School Funds
Historical data: See Table 41.

Table 43: Share of All Patient Activity in Teaching Hospitals
Historical data: *Data Book,* Association of American Medical Colleges, Data Series G.1.

Table 44: Research Spending on Noncommercial Biomedical Research
Historical data: National Health Accounts, *Health Care Financing Review,* Fall 1986.

Table 45: Medical Students and Medical Graduates
See Table 40.

Table 46: Applicants and Acceptances to Medical School
See Table 40.

Table 47: Research Spending on Noncommercial Biomedical Research
See Table 44.

Table 48: Medical School Income
See Table 41.

Table 49: Sources of Medical School Funds
See Table 42.

Table 50: Share of All Patient Activity in Teaching Hospitals
See Table 43.

Table 51: Academic Medical Centers: Comparative Summary of Scenarios
As previously referenced.

Table 52: Sources of Funds for Health Care
Historical data: National Health Accounts, *Health Care Financing Review,* Fall 1986.

Table 53: Market Share of Traditional Insurers
Historical data and forecasts estimates derived from BC/BS Panels.

Table 54: Concentration Ratio among Commercial Insurers
Historical data: Argus Chart of Health Insurance, various years, National Underwriter Company.

Table 55: Uninsured Population
Historical data: See sources for "Out of System" cited for Table 6.

Table 56: Net Cost of Insurance
Historical data: National Health Accounts, *Health Care Financing Review,* Fall 1986.

Table 57: Concentration Ratio among Commercial Insurers
See Table 54.

Table 58: Uninsured Population
See Table 55.

Table 59: Public Sector Spending
Historical data: National Health Accounts, *Health Care Financing Review,* Fall 1986.

Table 60: Government Health Spending
Historical data: See Table 59.

Table 61: Net Cost of Insurance
See Table 56.

Table 62: Insurers: Comparative Summary of Scenarios
As previously referenced.

Table 63: Hospital Costs
Historical data: American Hospital Association, *Hospital Statistics for Hospital Costs;* U.S. Department of Commerce, Bureau of Labor Statistics.

Table 64: Medical Care Variation
Chassin, M.R., et al., "Variations in the Use of Medical and Surgical Services by the Medical Population," *New England Journal of Medicine,* 1986, 314(5): 285-290.

Table 65: Infant Mortality Rates by Race
Historical data: National Center for Health Statistics.

Table 66: Prevention
Historical data: Louis Harris and Associates, *The Prevention Index,* 1986.

Table 67: Health Care Employment
Historical data: Kahl, A., and Clark, D.E., "Employment in Health Services Long-Term Trends and Projections," *Monthly Labor Review,* August 1986, pp. 17-36.

Table 68: Physicians' Services--Cost per Capita
Historical data: National Health Accounts, *Health Care Financing Review*.

Table 69: Hospital Costs
Historical data: American Hospital Association, *Hospital Statistics;* and BLS, *Employment and Earnings.*

Table 70: Program Administration and the Net Cost of Insurance
Historical data: National Health Accounts, *Health Care Financing Review*.

Table 71: Mean Fee for a Physician Visit
Historical data: American Medical Association, *Socioeconomic Monitoring System Surveys,* 1975-80, 1982-84, American Medical Association Periodic Surveys of Physicians.

Table 72: Medical Care Variation
See Table 64.

Table 73: Infant Mortality Rates by Race
Historical data: National Center for Health Statistics.

Table 74: Prevention
Historical data: Louis Harris and Associates, *The Prevention Index,* 1986.

Table 75: Health Care Employment
See Table 67.

Table 76: Public Policy: Comparative Summary of Scenarios
As previously referenced.

APPENDIX TABLES

Table B-1: List of Key Environmental Factors
IFTF.

Table E-1: Wild Cards
Expert interviews and PNO panels.

Table F-1: External Environment
As previously referenced.

Table F-2: Health Care System
As previously referenced.

Table F-3: Physicians
As previously referenced.

Table F-4: Hospitals
As previously referenced.

Table F-5: Academic Medical Centers
As previously referenced.

Table F-6: Insurers
As previously referred.